SLEEP WELL

Live Well

Strategies and solutions for getting the sleep you need for optimal health and happiness

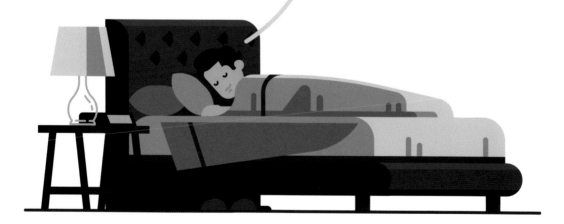

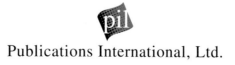

Publications International, Ltd.

Written by: Gary Gilles, M.A.

Consultant: Virgil D. Wooten, M.D.

Images: Shutterstock.com

Louis Weber, CEO
Publications International, Ltd.
8140 Lehigh Avenue
Morton Grove, IL 60053

ISBN: 978-1-68022-859-5

Manufactured in China.

8 7 6 5 4 3 2 1

Table of Contents

Introduction

SOUND SLEEP: FROM DREAM TO REALITY

Getting enough quality sleep is essential to physical, mental, and emotional health. Yet for too many people, a good night's sleep is like the Holy Grail—a priceless treasure they long for and seek but are too often unable to capture. If you're one of them, help is at hand.

Sleep Well, Live Well can help you unlock the door to dreamland and recapture the soothing, revitalizing benefits of deep, restful sleep. Within these pages, you'll discover the often-surprising factors and conditions that can prevent you from getting needed shut-eye. You'll be amazed at the many simple steps you can take to ensure better sleep. And you'll learn what to do when those simple steps aren't enough.

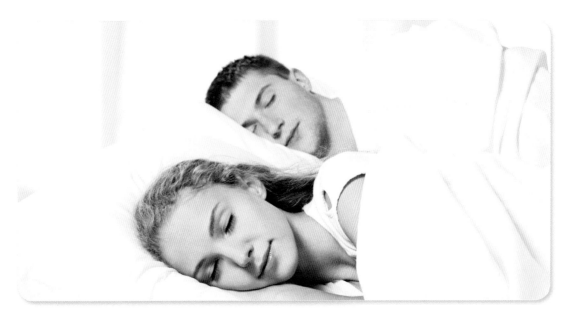

Chapter 1 provides an overview of that mysterious state we call sleep and why it's so important. You'll learn answers to such questions as: What actually happens when you sleep? How much sleep do you need? What happens when you are sleep-deprived? Why do some people sleep better than others?

Chapter 2 will teach you how to prepare for better sleep at night by making deliberate choices during the day. You'll learn about the connection between exercise and sleep, why getting natural sunlight in the morning is so important, what foods and beverages to avoid, and tips on managing stress.

Chapter 3 explores how to prepare your mind and body for sleep before bed. You'll learn relaxation techniques to employ and tips on how to avoid tossing and turning.

Chapter 4 covers how to make your sleep environment more conducive to restful slumber. Your bedroom should be a sanctuary free from potential sleep distractions such as TVs, computers, tablets, e-readers, and cell phones. This chapter offers tips on the best bedroom temperature, selecting the right mattress and pillow, and limiting the light and noise in your bedroom.

Chapter 5 explores common sleep disorders and problems such as sleep apnea, insomnia, narcolepsy, restless legs syndrome, and sleepwalking. It also includes a section on sleep disruptions caused by medical conditions.

Chapter 6 is about children and the sleep problems that can affect them. This includes descriptions of typical sleep patterns and of specific sleep disorders in children and adolescents.

Chapter 7 addresses the benefits and risks of prescription and over-the-counter sleep medications. You'll learn when they may be appropriate and how to use them safely.

Chapter 8 looks at complementary and alternative health approaches that may help you in your search for better sleep. You'll learn about melatonin and other supplements, herbal remedies, mindfulness and meditation, aromatherapy, acupuncture, massage, and yoga.

So if you're reading this through bleary eyes, don't despair. You can get on the path to a better night's sleep. Turning the page is your first step.

Chapter 1: The Importance of Sleep

SLEEP WAS LONG CONSID-ERED merely a block of time when the brain and body shut off. But we now know that brain and body functions remain active throughout sleep as we cycle through distinct stages. Each stage of sleep is linked to specific types of brain waves.

We need all stages of sleep to stay healthy and perform at our best. How well rested we are and how well we function the next day depend on our total sleep time and how much of the various stages of sleep we get each night.

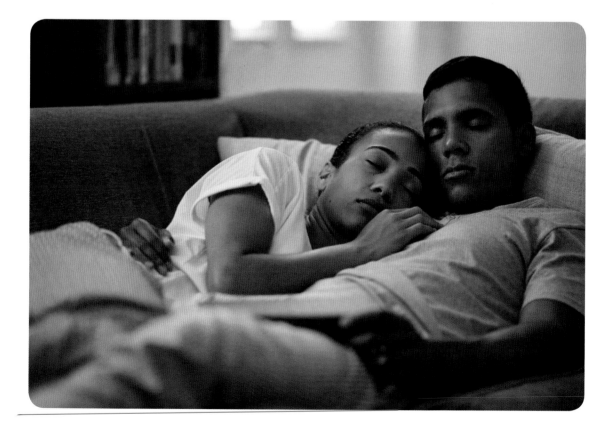

WHY DO WE SLEEP?

It should be obvious, right? Well it hasn't been so clear to some pretty smart people who have tried to figure it out. Listed here are some ideas that have been suggested over the years.

- Sleep is when the brain completely shuts down.
- Sleep is a response to boredom.
- Sleep occurs as a result of stomach vapors that cool the heart and block the brain's pores.

These and many other notions about why we sleep were proved wrong as researchers probed into the mysteries of sleep. Though many years of research have enlightened us to important aspects of sleep and why it's important, there is still much we don't know.

Here's a sampling of what we currently believe about why we sleep and about why sleep is so important:

• Sleep restores our mental energy. As we sleep, we tend to store and reorganize information we have accumulated throughout the day. (The brain doesn't shut down after all!) This regular mental housekeeping during sleep appears to enhance learning and creativity.

• Sleep is an important time when the body heals muscle tissue and restores itself. Our metabolic activity is at its lowest during deep sleep, providing an opportunity for the body to rebuild and heal. This is crucial both during the growth years of childhood and during adult life.

• During sleep, our brain waves slow down considerably compared to our waking state. This slowing of brain waves creates a combination of light and deep sleep that cycles repeatedly through the night. Our degree of refreshment the next day depends on how these cycles play out while we sleep.

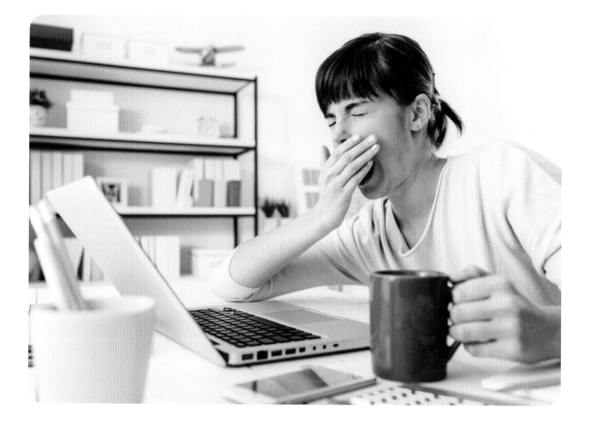

THE TOLL OF TOO LITTLE SLEEP

The most obvious negative consequence of sleep deprivation is daytime sleepiness. We all go through occasional periods when we get less sleep than we need. When we catch up on our sleep and return to getting the needed amount of rest each night, the sleepiness and fatigue disappear. But chronic sleep deprivation causes more than fatigue. It can lead to a variety of serious physical, mental, and social problems and even increase the risk of death.

EMOTIONAL EFFECTS

If you have gone without sleep for any length of time, you know that you can become irritable, impatient, or even aggressive when you are tired. Insufficient sleep is linked to poor behavior and trouble with relationships, especially among children and teens. Even a small degree of sleep deprivation can contribute to depression or anxiety. People who are chronically sleep deprived are more likely to become depressed.

MENTAL-FUNCTIONING EFFECTS

We need sleep to think clearly, react quickly, and create memories. Anyone who has pulled an "all-nighter" studying for an exam or keeping a vigil at the hospital knows the muddled sensation of a tired mind. One of the immediate consequences of sleep deprivation is poor concentration and lack of sound judgment. Cutting back by even one hour can make it tough to focus the next day and can slow response time. Studies find that lack of sleep leads to faulty decision-making, more risk taking, and slower reaction time. This can result in lower performance at school or on the job and an increased risk for a car accident.

PHYSICAL EFFECTS

Sleep is critical for good health. Not getting enough quality sleep on a regular basis increases the risk of developing high blood pressure and other cardiovascular problems, diabetes, depression, and obesity.

Evidence is growing that sleep is a powerful regulator of appetite, energy use, and weight control. Studies find that the less people sleep, the more likely they are to be overweight or obese, to develop diabetes, and to prefer eating foods that are high in calories and carbohydrates.

Another consequence of sleep deprivation is a compromised immune system. Even a modest reduction in sleep has been shown to affect immune response. If you are sleep deprived, you are at greater risk for flu, colds, and other infections. Fortunately, the immune system will bounce back quickly if you get the consistent rest you need.

ACCIDENTS

It should come as little surprise that a sleep-deprived person is also more prone to accidents. Perhaps the greatest danger is a sleep-deprived person operating heavy equipment or a motor vehicle. Research from the AAA Foundation for Traffic Safety shows that approximately 25 percent of subjects interviewed admit to falling asleep at the wheel of a car or truck at least once over the past year. And falling asleep at the wheel isn't the only danger with driving drowsy. Like alcohol, lack of sleep slows reaction time. This makes it harder to respond quickly to a suddenly breaking car, a sharp curve in the road, or other dangerous situations. An estimated seven percent of all crashes and 16.5 percent of fatal crashes involve a drowsy driver.

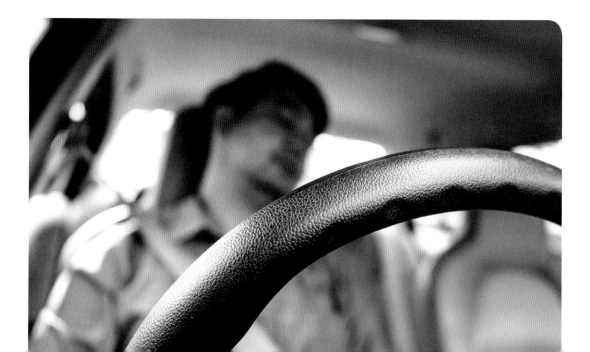

DROWSY DRIVING

Classic symptoms of drowsy driving:

- You have trouble keeping your eyes open or focused.
- You can't stop yawning.
- You can't remember driving the past few miles.
- You miss road signs or drive past your usual turn.
- You find yourself drifting out of your lane or tailgating.

Having even one of these symptoms is a sign that you need to stop and get some sleep before driving again.

Tips to avoid drowsy driving:

- Be well rested before hitting the road.
- Avoid driving between midnight and 7 a.m.
- Don't drive alone.
- Schedule frequent breaks on long trips.
- Don't drink alcohol.
- Don't count on caffeine.

ARE YOU SLEEP DEPRIVED?

Take this short quiz to help determine whether you are sleep deprived. Mark true (T) or false (F) for each.

1. I need an alarm clock in order to wake up at the correct time. _____
2. I hit the snooze button several times to get more sleep. _____
3. I struggle to get out of bed in the morning. _____
4. I often fall asleep at inappropriate times during the day. _____
5. I feel tired, irritable, and stressed out during the week. _____
6. I often fall asleep in boring meetings or warm rooms. _____
7. I often need a nap to get through the day. _____
8. I have trouble focusing during the day. _____
9. I often fall asleep after consuming a small amount of alcohol. _____
10. I often feel drowsy while driving. _____
11. I often fall asleep within five minutes of getting into bed. _____
12. I often sleep in extra hours on weekend mornings. _____

If you answered "true" to at least three of these statements, there is a good chance you are sleep deprived.

DEVELOPING A RHYTHM

Years ago, before the invention of electricity, people went to bed shortly after the sun went down. Sure, it sounds boring, but there was a predictable rhythm to life that was dictated by sunshine and darkness. People worked hard during the day and slept well and long at night. But in modern times, we tend to move to a different beat. Our frenetic "always on the go" lifestyle has disrupted the rhythm of sleep that humans had grown accustomed to over centuries. Sleep now competes against work; personal, family, and social commitments; and a host of entertainment options, almost all of which are no longer restricted to daylight hours. This is not necessarily a bad turn of events, but it creates challenges for us in terms of getting the rest we need.

Fortunately, we have a built-in body clock that attempts to keep us in step with a normal 24-hour cycle of waking and sleeping. This body clock is often referred to as the circadian rhythm. The term *circadian*, translated from Latin, simply means "about a day." It is our body's natural way of trying to regulate not only our sleep patterns but a variety of other bodily processes, including digestion, elimination, growth, renewal of cells, and body temperature. When we work with our body's natural cycle, we can greatly improve not only our sleep but also our overall health.

When we fight against that cycle, on the other hand, our sleep, waking performance, and health can suffer.

Take, for example, a woman we'll call Diane. Diane is self-employed and works from home. She doesn't have a set time for going to bed or getting up each day; it pretty much depends on what she's doing on any particular day. She often works late into the night on various projects, finally retiring at 3 or 4 a.m. Following late-nighters,

she tends to sleep in until about noon. Other nights she's so tired from her late-night routine that she goes to bed at 8 p.m. and sleeps for 12 hours. She finds that at least two or three days a week she needs a 30-minute "power nap" during the afternoon to get her through the day. Diane is wreaking havoc with her body clock with this inconsistent wake-sleep schedule. There is no rhythm to speak of. It's not surprising, then, that she often does not sleep well when she does hit the bed. She's not giving her body a chance to develop a predictable 24-hour rhythm that could better equip her for productive work during the day and restful sleep at night.

This is one of the main reasons sleep experts recommend going to bed and rising at the same time each day, even on weekends. It helps keep the circadian rhythm working in your favor. Different ages, sleep needs, and lifestyle patterns require different wake-sleep rhythms. The goal is to find what works best for you and stick with it. (Chapter 5 talks more about working with your body clock when it needs resetting.)

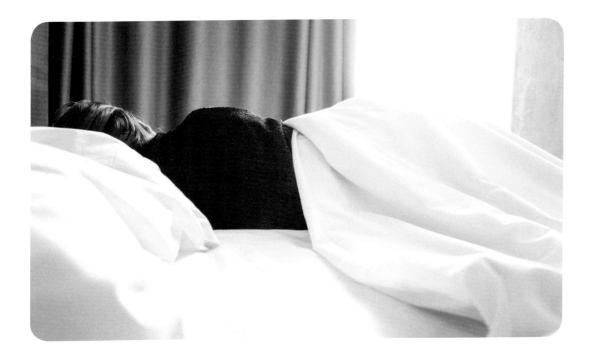

WHAT HAPPENS DURING SLEEP?

A lot more than you probably realize. It was widely believed until about midway through the twentieth century that there was only one type of sleep. Whether you got one hour or ten hours of sleep, it was the same garden variety. With the help of modern technology, we now know that not all sleep is the same. The two main types of sleep are rapid eye movement (REM) sleep and non-REM (NREM) sleep.

REM sleep gets its name from the distinctive shifting of the eyes that occurs during this state. In non-REM sleep, the distinctive rapid eye movements are absent. Non-REM sleep is further divided into four stages. You repeatedly pass through REM and the four stages of NREM for different lengths of time during a typical night's sleep.

SLEEP MONITORING

You might wonder how researchers can accurately tell you what is happening in your mind and body while you doze. Scientists developed a test called polysomnography (also called a sleep study), which monitors your brain waves, eye movements, heart rate, airflow, breathing pattern, body position, limb movement, and blood-oxygen level while you sleep. Electrodes (small adhesive patches with wires attached) are placed on your scalp and other parts of your body to record this activity. The results give sleep specialists an accurate picture of what is happening in your body, because different stages of sleep are marked by distinct brain waves and physical responses. See chapter 5 for more about sleep studies.

A sleep study performed during an overnight visit to a sleep center can help diagnose disorders such as sleep apnea.

SLEEP STATES

When you sleep, you cycle through five distinct phases—stage 1, 2, 3, 4, and rapid eye movement (REM) sleep. The following page has a brief summary of what goes on during these sleep stages.

Stage 1 (non-REM) This first stage of non-REM sleep is where you transition from wakefulness to sleep. It lasts only five to ten minutes for most people. During this period of very light sleep, your eyes move slowly beneath their lids, your heart rate and breathing begin to slow, and your muscles relax. You can be awakened easily out of this stage of sleep, and if this happens, you may feel as if you haven't slept at all. Most people only spend about five percent of their total sleeping time in stage 1.

Stage 2 (non-REM) In this stage, eye movements cease, brain waves slow (although occasional bursts of greater brain activity occur), body temperature and metabolic rate drop, and breathing and heart rate are slow and steady. During this stage, you can still be awakened easily. Most people spend about 45 to 50 percent of their total sleep time in stage 2.

Stages 3 and 4 (non-REM) As you drift into stage 3 and then stage 4—considered deep, more restorative sleep phases—your brain waves become large and very slow, your muscles go limp, your heart and breathing rates decrease further, and your blood pressure drops. At the same time, hormones are released that promote tissue growth and repair. Waking you from these stages of sleep can be difficult, and you may experience a few moments of grogginess before becoming alert. Most people spend 20 to 25 percent of their total sleep time in stages 3 and 4, mostly during the first half of the night.

REM Sleep It is in the REM sleep state that you do most of your dreaming. In REM, your heart rate, blood pressure, and breathing become irregular, and your eyes involuntarily dart back and forth rapidly, but the muscles in your arms and legs are paralyzed. REM sleep is considered a deep and restorative state that reenergizes both body and brain and is necessary for higher brain function during waking hours. Sleepers in REM stage are hard to awaken. Most people spend about 25 percent of their total sleep time in REM sleep.

HOW THE SLEEP STATES FIT TOGETHER

As you go from stage 1 to stage 4 of NREM sleep, your brain and body become increasingly more relaxed. Once you reach REM sleep, however, both brain and body functions switch gears. Your heart rate and breathing speed up, and your fingers, face, and legs may twitch. These responses are indicators that your brain is in a more active state.

Normally you cycle in and out of REM sleep throughout the night. Because it typically takes 90 minutes or so to go from awake to the end of the fourth stage of NREM sleep, the first REM period usually begins about 90 minutes after you doze off and lasts about ten minutes. Subsequent REM periods

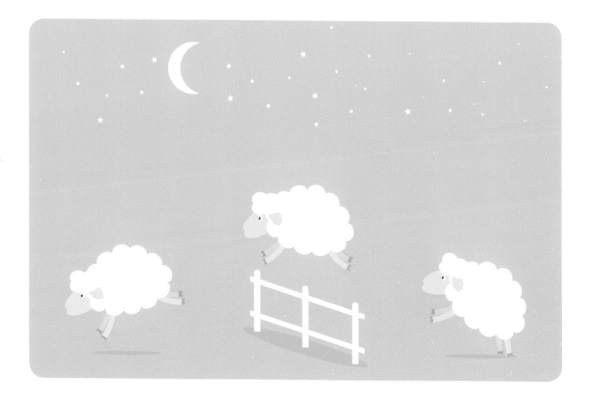

gradually increase in length as the night wears on, with the final period lasting 40 to 60 minutes.

Between REM periods, you return to NREM stage 2 and work your way back to REM. Over the course of the night, you cycle through these stages four to six times, depending on how long you sleep. If you awaken during the night, it is usually when you are moving from the end of a REM cycle back to NREM stage 2, and you typically fall back to sleep immediately without even realizing you were awake.

It is this cycling, and especially the time spent in REM sleep, that determines how rested you feel when you wake up. If you don't get a long-enough period of undisturbed sleep, you won't spend enough time cycling through the sleep stages, and you will likely feel tired and unrefreshed when you get up. The body can compensate for short periods of sleep deprivation, but frequent or extended episodes of diminished sleep create a sleep debt that can have a variety of detrimental effects.

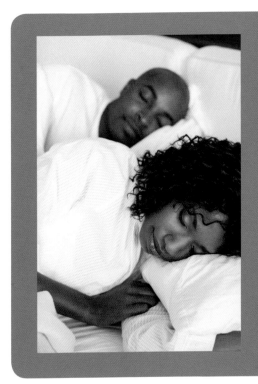

EVERYBODY HAS A DREAM

Many people don't think they dream at night because they don't remember their dreams. But provided they enter REM sleep, everyone spends up to two hours dreaming each night. Most people average about four dreams per night, each lasting roughly 20 minutes. We can dream in all stages of sleep but dreams are usually most vivid in REM sleep.

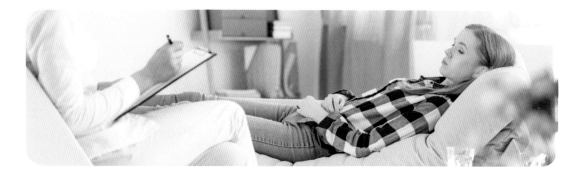

DREAM ON

Through the ages, many people and cultures have attempted to understand and assign meaning to dreams. Perhaps the best-known dream interpreter was Sigmund Freud. He believed that dreams revealed psychological needs and wishes in a person's life that were often unconscious. While the exact purpose of dreaming isn't known, most modern sleep experts believe that dreaming is an important way we process our emotions and life experiences that happen during waking hours. For instance, if you watch a scary movie right before bed, there's a good chance some of the images and emotion you experience during the movie will find their way into your dreams that night.

WHAT MAKES YOU SLEEP?

Your eventual need for sleep is due in part to two substances your body produces—adenosine and melatonin. While you're awake, the level of adenosine in your body continues to rise. The increasing level of adenosine signals a shift toward sleep. While you sleep, your body breaks down adenosine. The other substance that helps you sleep is the hormone melatonin. When it gets dark, your internal biological clock triggers your body to produce melatonin, which prepares your brain and body for sleep. As melatonin is released, you feel increasingly drowsy.

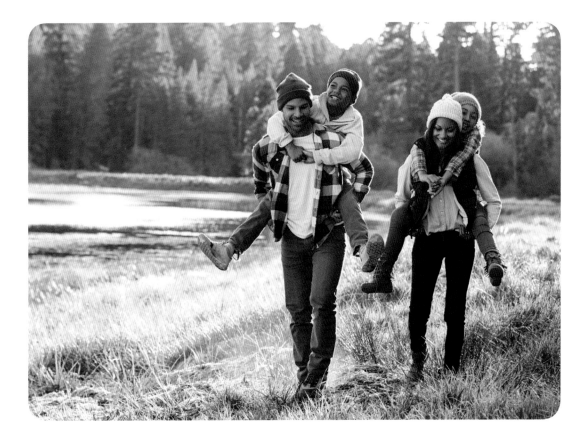

HOW MUCH SLEEP DO YOU NEED?

Although sleep needs vary somewhat among individuals, there is a certain minimum amount of sleep humans require. Research indicates that to perform adequately at home and on the job—in other words, without falling asleep at the wheel, making dumb mistakes due to tiredness, or being cranky and impatient with others—and also to avoid the increased health risks of chronic sleep deficiency, most adults need seven to eight hours of sleep each night. Some adults called "short sleepers" naturally require less than six hours of sleep at night. At the other end of the spectrum are "long sleepers" who need nine or more hours of sleep per night.

The amount of sleep you need depends on your age, level of activity, emotional state, and other factors. Regardless of your normal sleep needs, you may need additional sleep when you are recovering from a serious infection, illness, or surgery. You may also require more rest when mourning the loss of a loved one, going through a divorce or breakup, or experiencing some other unusual stress.

Yet in America today, the average adult sleeps fewer than seven hours a night. More than one-third of adults report that, at least a few times each month, daytime sleepiness is so severe that their work, interactions with others, and driving ability suffer. Children and adolescents are also getting less sleep than recommended. Lack of sleep may have a direct effect on children's health, behavior, and development.

RECOMMENDED SLEEP DURATIONS

The National Sleep Foundation recommends the following sleep durations:

Newborns (0–3 months old):	14–17 hours
Infants (4–11 months old):	12–15 hours
Toddlers (1–2 years old):	11–14 hours
Preschoolers (3–5 years old):	10–13 hours
School-aged (6–13 years old):	9–11 hours
Teenagers (14–17 years old):	8–10 hours
Adults (18–64 years old):	7–9 hours
Older adults (≥ 65 years old):	7–8 hours

AGE AND SLEEP

So far, our discussion has focused primarily on the sleep needs and patterns of average adults. For children, adolescents, and, to a lesser extent, seniors, these patterns and needs can be quite different.

CHILDREN

You may have noticed that infants sleep a lot—but not always at the times their parents want them to. During the first few months of life, an infant has two basic jobs: eating and sleeping. An infant typically sleeps an average of 16 to 18 hours each day and needs every bit of it for proper growth and development. Infants tend to sleep in four- to five-hour blocks of time and wake when they are hungry. The natural sleep-wake rhythm of infants is weighted heavily toward sleep. So in a 24-hour cycle, an infant will sleep two-thirds or more of that time. In contrast, an adult on average sleeps only one-third of that total daily cycle.

As a child develops, their sleep time gradually decreases. At six months, the average sleep time is 14 hours; at age two, that has dropped further to around 12.5 hours. By the time a child reaches age six, sleep time is reduced to about 11 hours, and naps are often no longer needed.

During a child's elementary school years, sleep patterns begin to more closely resemble those of adults. Grade-schoolers sleep more deeply in certain phases of sleep, which indicates their brains are maturing in their ability to store and process information from the day.

ADOLESCENTS

Most teenagers have a love-hate relationship with sleep. They want to stay up way too late on school nights—or every night, in some instances. Then on a Saturday or a school holiday, they prefer to hibernate in bed for most of the day. It's not uncommon for a wary parent to sneak into their teen's room at 3:00 p.m. to listen for signs of breathing. While this pattern of sleep may be confusing to parents, there seem to be some good reasons for this erratic sleep behavior.

Research indicates that this tendency toward being a night owl may have a biological origin in adolescents. The bodily changes they experience in puberty reset their sleep-wake clock so they are not ready to fall asleep until 11 p.m. or later. Of course, the problem is not so much with staying up late as it is with getting up early for school. The average teen needs somewhere between eight and ten hours of sleep a night, but few get that much on a regular basis. Most adolescents get seven or fewer hours of sleep a night. The National Sleep Foundation reports that 60 percent of teens feel tired during the day and 15 percent report falling asleep in class during the past year.

adults. As people age, however, nighttime sleep tends to be shorter, lighter, and interrupted by more awakenings. Older people also spend less time in the deep, restful stage of sleep. Poor lifestyle habits and chronic illness can also disrupt sleep.

It used to be thought that the internal body clock of older people required them to get less sleep. Research has shown this notion to be false. It is true that seniors tend to rise earlier in the morning and become sleepy in the afternoon. This is due to the internal body clock setting itself to a different rhythm as we age. Social factors, such as going to bed early out of boredom, and medical illnesses and medications that cause fatigue and sleepiness, may also cause earlier bedtimes and therefore earlier morning awakenings.

SENIORS

Answer true or false about the following statement: Seniors don't need as much sleep as they did when they were younger. Most people would say "true." And most people would be wrong. There is no evidence that seniors need less sleep than younger adults. Older adults require the same seven to eight hours of sleep as other

WHY DO SOME PEOPLE SLEEP BETTER THAN OTHERS?

If you can stay awake for the answer, you'll discover that you're not alone in asking that question. It's estimated that over 100 million Americans are chronically sleep-deprived. There are two main reasons for this. The first involves lifestyle habits.

LIFESTYLE HABITS

Ever since short-sleeper Thomas Edison invented the light bulb, we have been staying up later into the night. But he doesn't deserve all of the blame. Over the years, we have evolved into a 24/7 culture that pushes limits. As work, family, entertainment, and a seemingly infinite number of responsibilities and experiences tug at our limited time, we tend to steal time from the most available source: our sleeping hours.

The National Sleep Foundation regularly conducts surveys to

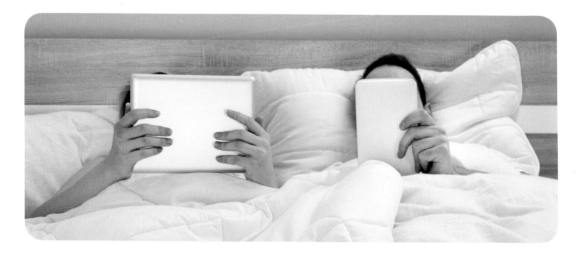

measure sleep habits of Americans. Findings show that nearly two-thirds of adults do not get the recommended eight hours of sleep per night. Of course, some of these folks are short sleepers and don't need eight hours, but many do need that much and are not getting it. One-third of the respondents reported getting less than seven hours of sleep each night. And one-quarter claim that they are so sleepy during the day that their fatigue interferes with daily activities. The practical translation of these statistics: There are a lot of chronically tired people walking around.

A common trick many use in an effort to catch up on their sleep is to spend more time sleeping on the weekends. While this may help somewhat in the short-term, it rarely balances the books. Instead, the sleep that is lost accumulates over time into what is called sleep debt.

You create a sleep debt when you "borrow" hours that you really need for sleep and use them for something else, often with the assumption that you'll try to "repay" them at a later time. Say, for

example, that a fellow named John knows he functions best on eight hours of sleep. But he works two jobs and finds that he can't get everything done without staying up later at night. He averages about 6.5 hours of sleep a night. So the difference between the sleep he needs to be alert and fully rested and what he actually gets is 1.5 hours a night. By the end of the workweek, he has "borrowed" 7.5 hours from his sleep account (1.535 days). In an effort to make up for lost dozing time, he sleeps about nine hours each on Saturday and Sunday. So John makes a "deposit" of two hours back into his sleep account over the weekend. But this still leaves him short 5.5 hours for the week. So while a little extra sleep on the weekend helps, John never truly catches up on his sleep and feels chronically tired. He is tired so much of the time that he has begun to feel this is normal for him. The only way John can erase the debt is to change his sleep routine to get the sleep he needs on a regular basis.

SLEEP DISORDERS

Those who are tired because of lifestyle habits tend to cheat themselves of sleep. But those who suffer from a sleep disorder feel they are being robbed of their sleep by a force beyond their control. More than 70 different sleep disorders affect millions of people. People with chronic health problems (currently 45 percent of the population) are among those most prone to having a sleep disorder. Sleep disruptions may also be caused by pain, disability, medication, or another source.

COMMON SIGNS OF A SLEEP DISORDER

- You consistently need more than 30 minutes to fall asleep each night.
- You wake up several times each night and then having trouble falling back to sleep, or you wake up too early in the morning.
- You often feel sleepy during the day, take frequent naps, or fall asleep unexpectedly at inappropriate times during the day.
- Your bed partner says that you loudly snore, snort, gasp, make choking sounds, or stop breathing for short periods when sleeping.
- You have creeping, tingling, or crawling feelings in your legs or arms that are relieved by moving or massaging them, especially at bedtime.
- You have vivid, dreamlike experiences while falling asleep.
- You feel like you cannot move when you first wake up.
- Your bed partner says that you often jerk your legs or arms during sleep.
- You have episodes of sudden muscle weakness when you are angry or fearful, or when you laugh.
- You don't feel rested despite getting 8 or more hours of sleep at night.
- You require stimulants to stay awake during the day.

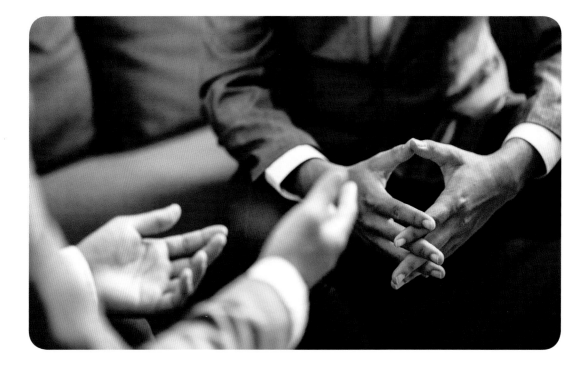

WHEN TO SEEK HELP

You should seek medical help if your sleep problem persists for three weeks or more. Of course, if the problem is severe—if you're getting fewer than three hours of sleep each night, for example—it may be advisable to consult a physician sooner. You should also contact your doctor if you've been told that you snore loudly and/or seem to temporarily stop breathing during sleep; these symptoms may indicate sleep apnea, a condition that can be life-threatening.

Problems with daytime sleepiness also demand attention. The most common cause of daytime sleepiness is not getting enough sleep at night. If you regularly allow yourself sufficient time for sleep but still find yourself drifting off at inappropriate times (such as at work, school, or when driving), seek medical attention as soon as possible. Such significant daytime sleepiness is a serious symptom that should never be ignored.

If you decide to see a doctor, who should it be? Usually, it's reasonable to start with your primary doctor. He or she will likely take a history of your sleep problem, conduct a physical exam, and order routine blood tests to rule out most medical problems. Should the results of these tests be negative, a referral to a sleep specialist may be the next step.

You should consider several factors when looking for a sleep specialist. First, make sure the doctor has the proper credentials. Sleep specialists should be board certified in sleep medicine. Sleep doctors often have training in a second area: psychiatry, neurology, or internal medicine.

If your doctor refers you to a sleep center for diagnosis, the American Academy of Sleep Medicine (AASM) should accredit the center. The AASM is the professional organization for sleep medicine in the United States. Each accredited laboratory is inspected to ensure it meets standards set by the AASM. Sleep centers that are not accredited may or may not adhere to guidelines of the AASM. Be wary of a recommendation for sleep studies performed in the home. These tests have serious limitations and are often performed by those with inadequate training.

You'll gain more insight into particular sleep disorders and their treatments in chapter 5.

GET IT IN WRITING

By now, you may think you know whether you are getting enough sleep on a nightly basis. But consider these specific questions.

- How many hours of sleep do you average each night?
- How many hours do you think you need to function at your best physically and mentally?
- What is your sleep debt per week?
- How many times per night do you typically awaken from sleep?

Most people, when asked these questions, can only give approximate numbers. But the answers to these questions are very important for you to know if you want to correct current sleeping problems. The best way to begin is to keep what's known as a sleep diary.

A sleep diary will show you exactly what is occurring with your sleep habits. There are many variations of sleep diaries. Page 31 shows one simple format that only takes a few minutes to fill out each day. You can draw or make your own chart by following the sample format.

Virtually all sleep clinics instruct their patients to use sleep diaries at some point to gather important information about sleep habits before they begin treatment for problems. The answers you log in your sleep diary might surprise you! You might think you're getting eight hours of sleep, only for the diary to reveal that while you spend eight hours in bed, you only get seven hours of sleep because of bathroom breaks or other matters. That sleep debt accumulates quickly!

TO USE THE SAMPLE SLEEP DIARY:

1. In the upper left-hand corner of your diary page, under "Sleep goal," record what you believe to be the number of sleep hours you need each night to feel your best.

2. When you go to bed, mentally note the time.

3. In the morning, record this information:
   - Time you got into bed
   - Approximate time it took you to fall asleep

- Number of times you awoke during the night and why
- How long it took you to go back to sleep after being awake
- Time you got up

4. Subtract or add actual hours of sleep from your nightly sleep goal. Include time awake during the night.

5. At week's end, tally the "+/- sleep needed" column.

SAMPLE SLEEP DIARY

Sleep goal	Time I went to bed	Time it took to fall asleep	No. of awaken-ings per night/ reasons	How long awake each night	Time I got up in the morning	Total sleep time	+/- sleep needed
Mon.							
Tue.							
Wed.							
Thur.							
Fri.							
Sat.							
Sun.							
Totals							

Chapter 2: Prepare for Sleep All Day

OFTEN, WE ARE OUR OWN worst enemies when it comes to getting needed sleep. Take the case of Henry. After racing all day at work, he continues his relentless pace in his non-work hours, trying to squeeze in all of the things he needs or wants to do. At some late hour he gets hit with fatigue. It's the first time since awakening early that morning that he has even thought about sleep. And that's a major mistake. Because now, deciding it is time to go to bed, he assumes that putting a toothbrush in his mouth, peeling the covers back, and closing his eyes will perform a magical spell that will catapult him into deep, refreshing sleep.

But sound sleep is not what Henry typically experiences. After driving his body and mind at 80 miles per hour for the entire day and evening, he slams on the brakes and rolls into bed. While his intention is to sleep, his mind and body are not ready. He's taken no time or effort to prepare himself for a good night's sleep. But should he?

The answer is a definite yes, despite the fact that most people don't. That lack of preparation could have something to do with the fact that over half the population of the United States complains of sleep problems.

From the moment you wake up in the morning, you face decisions that can affect how well you sleep at night. Making wise choices throughout the day can help you sleep soundly at night and awaken with renewed energy. This chapter is designed to help you prepare yourself for a good night's rest all day long.

EXERCISE TO SLEEP BETTER

Most people claim that they don't exercise on a regular basis because they are too tired. Perhaps that has something to do with sleep habits. If there was a "best intention never acted on" competition, exercise would probably win. The reason we intend to exercise is that we know it's good for us. Regular exercise improves heart health and blood pressure, builds bone and muscle, helps combat stress and muscle tension, and can even improve mood. Add one more benefit: sound sleep. Did you know that exercise can help you sleep sounder and longer and feel more awake during the day? It's true. But the key is found in the type of exercise you choose and the time you participate in it during the day.

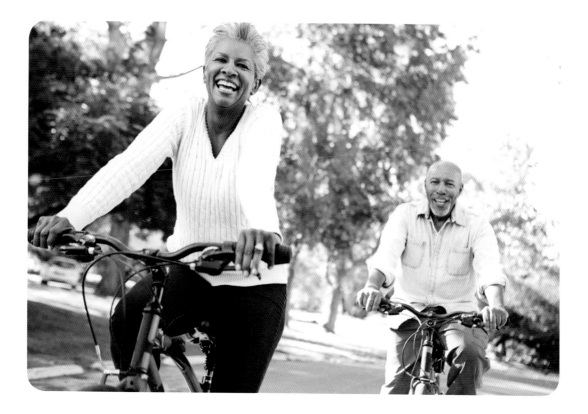

TIMING AND TYPE OF EXERCISE

What time of the day do you think exercise would best help you sleep? Morning? Afternoon? Evening? Right before bed?

Exercising vigorously right before bed or within about three hours of your bedtime can actually make it harder to fall asleep. This surprises many people; it's often thought that a good workout before bed helps you feel more tired. In actuality, vigorous exercise right before bed stimulates your heart, brain, and muscles— the opposite of what you want at bedtime. It also raises your body temperature right before bed, which is not what you want.

Morning exercise can relieve stress and improve mood. These effects can indirectly improve sleep, no doubt. To get a more direct sleep-promoting benefit from morning exercise, however, you can couple it with exposure to outdoor light. Being exposed to natural light in the morning, whether you're exercising or not, can improve your sleep at night by reinforcing your body's sleep-wake cycle.

When it comes to having a direct effect on getting a good night's sleep, it's vigorous exercise in the late afternoon or early evening that appears most beneficial. That's because it raises your body temperature above normal a few hours before bed, allowing it to start falling just as you're getting

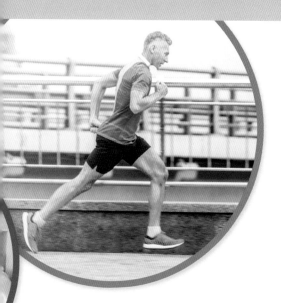

The type of vigorous workout we're talking about is a cardiovascular workout. That means you engage in some activity in which you keep your heart rate up and your muscles pumping continuously for at least 20 minutes. Although strength-training, stretching, yoga, and other methods of exercise are beneficial, none match the sleep-enhancing benefits of cardiovascular exercise.

ready for bed. This decrease in body temperature appears to be a trigger that helps ease you into sleep (see the Exercise-Sleep Connection sidebar on page 36).

Try to schedule at least 20 minutes of vigorous exercise three or four times a week. Choose whatever activity you enjoy. Walk to and from work, or walk the dog. Jog, swim,

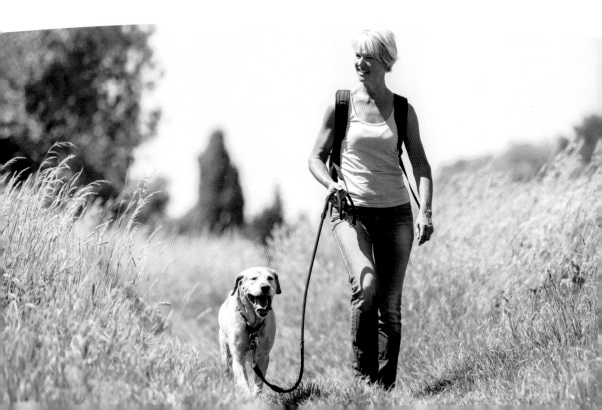

THE EXERCISE-SLEEP CONNECTION

Everyone's body temperature naturally goes up slightly in the daytime and back down at night, reaching its low just before dawn. Decreasing body temperature seems to be a trigger, signaling the body that it's time to sleep. Vigorous exercise temporarily raises the body temperature as much as two degrees. Twenty or 30 minutes of aerobic exercise is sufficient to keep the body temperature at this higher level for a period of four to five hours, after which it drops lower than if you hadn't exercised. This lower body temperature is what helps you sleep better. So if you exercise five to six hours before going to bed, you will be attempting to sleep at the same time your temperature is beginning to go down. That's the best way to maximize exercise's beneficial effects on sleep.

bike, ski, jump rope, dance, or play tennis—just make it part of your routine. If you have any serious medical conditions, are very overweight, or haven't exercised in years, talk to your doctor about your plans for exercising before you begin. Be sure to start exercising slowly, gradually increasing your workout time and intensity, so you don't get sidelined by injury. Remember, regular exercise can help you feel, look, and sleep better.

BRIGHTEN YOUR MORNING

Light tells the brain it is time to wake up. That's probably obvious to anyone who has had to turn on a light in the middle of the night and then has had trouble getting back to sleep. What may not be so obvious is that exposure to light at other times, particularly in the early morning, can actually help you sleep at night.

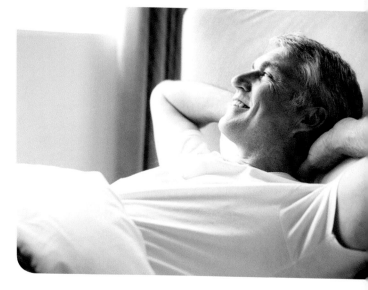

How does morning light improve sleep? The light helps to regulate your biological clock and keep it on track. This internal clock is located in the brain and keeps time not all that much differently from your wristwatch. There does, however, appear to be a kind of forward drift built into the brain. By staying up later and, more importantly, getting up later, you enforce that drift, which means you may find you have trouble getting to sleep and waking up when you need to. To counter this forward drift, you need to reset your clock each day, so that it stays compatible with the earth's 24-hour daily rhythm—and with your daily schedule. Exposing yourself to light in the morning appears to accomplish this resetting. Research has shown that people who are deprived of light for long periods of time (and so do not have their biological clocks reset) experience dramatic changes in their sleep, temperature, and hormone cycles. Although you probably won't be deprived of light for an extended period, getting less morning light than you need may make it more difficult for you to fall asleep and wake up at your preferred times.

Many factors can affect our biological clock, but light appears to be the most important. The timing of exposure is crucial; the body clock is most responsive to sunlight in the early morning, between 6:00 and 8:30 a.m. Exposure to sunlight later does not provide the same benefit. The type of light also matters, as does the length of exposure. Direct sunlight outdoors for at least 30 minutes produces the most benefit. The indoor lighting in a typical

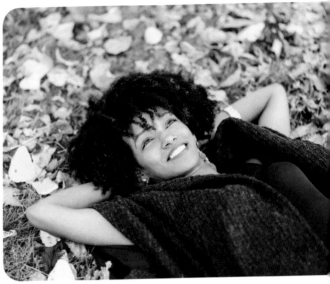

home, school, or office has little effect. Specially designed light boxes and visors that simulate sunlight are available. (They are often prescribed to treat seasonal affective disorder, or SAD, a form of depression that tends to occur seasonally, during the darker winter months.) Still, a half hour in front of even the most powerful light box does not provide as much light therapy as does a half hour outside on even an overcast day—natural light is best.

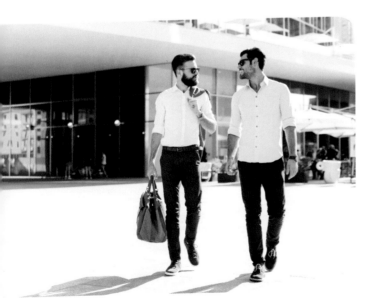

LIGHT THERAPY

If you're battling insomnia but can't consistently expose yourself to outdoor light in the morning, you may want to try light therapy with artificial light. This involves sitting near an artificial-light box that mimics natural outdoor light and has a similar effect on your biological clock. Light therapy is most effective when you have the proper combination of light intensity, duration, and timing.

- **Intensity:** The intensity of a light box is recorded in lux, which is a measure of the amount of light you receive. You need a 10,000-lux light box to regulate your rhythm.

- **Duration:** Light therapy with a 10,000-lux light box typically involves daily sessions of about 20–30 minutes. Check the manufacturer's guidelines and follow your doctor's instructions.

- **Timing:** For most people, light therapy is most effective when it's done early in the morning, after you first wake up. Your doctor can help you determine the light therapy schedule that works best.

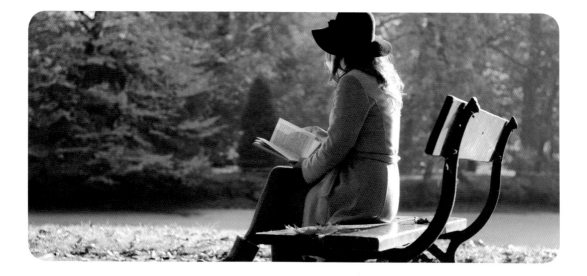

MANAGE STRESS

If you moved into a new neighborhood only to discover that it was plagued by smelly smoke from a nearby factory, you would likely be annoyed or angry at first. But after several weeks, you probably wouldn't notice it as much. You would become conditioned to the smell despite the fact that it may not be terribly healthy for you. A similar phenomenon can occur when we experience stress on an ongoing basis. We may be so bombarded with daily stress—in the form of hurried schedules, family commitments, traffic jams, and the like—that we become accustomed to it. We may not even realize how stressed we are until we're faced with a breakdown or an emergency—a "last straw." But such constant exposure to stress can make it difficult to get needed

ARE YOU STRESSED OUT?

Here are some classic symptoms of stress:

- Rapid heart rate
- Sweating palms, armpits
- Clenched jaw
- Tight muscles in the neck, shoulders, back
- Hunched, drooping shoulders
- Tight feeling in the chest
- Intense look on the face
- Shallow breathing
- Irritability, short temper

sleep and can compromise our overall health.

It's important to dispel the myth that you can avoid stress. If you breathe, you are going to encounter life situations that bring stress. Since you can't avoid it, the best option is to learn to manage it. One key to managing stress is assessing what you have control over and what you don't. For instance, if your boss has set an unrealistic deadline for a project, you may have little or no control over changing that. But you do have control over how you respond to that deadline. And your response to a given situation is what you want to focus on as you seek to manage stress. You can choose to do certain things and not others. This ability to choose puts you in control and gives you the ability to make the situation work for you.

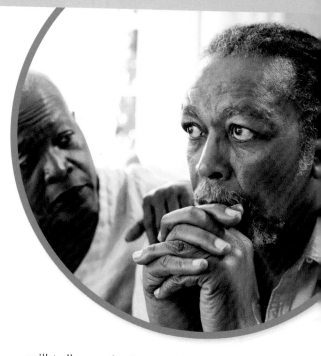

Professional therapists who specialize in stress reduction will tell you that your body is the best guide to determining when you are feeling stressed. If you pay attention to how you feel both physically and emotionally, you can often intervene before stress begins to interfere with sleep.

What does stress management during the day have to do with sleeping well at night? Plenty. Have you ever had the unpleasant experience of crawling into bed exhausted, wanting to put a terrible day behind you, and spending the next few hours tossing and turning as you go over every detail of your day? That is stress at work on your mind. All of those emotions

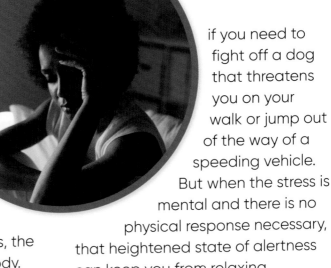

and thoughts throughout the day that were not dealt with at the time can work their way to the surface in the quiet of night.

In addition, the more you dwell on the upsetting events, the greater the effect on your body. When it senses stress, the brain sends a message to the body to release hormones that heighten alertness and prepare it for action. This is known as the fight-or-flight response. It's a beneficial reaction if you need to fight off a dog that threatens you on your walk or jump out of the way of a speeding vehicle. But when the stress is mental and there is no physical response necessary, that heightened state of alertness can keep you from relaxing enough to sleep. By learning to deal with stressors in your life more immediately during the day, you are less likely to be kept awake by them at night.

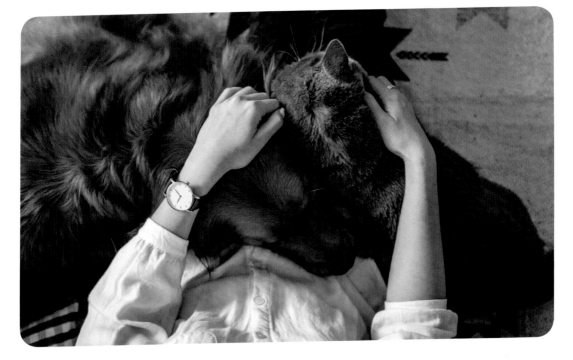

10 WAYS TO LOWER STRESS IN FIVE MINUTES OR LESS

1. Sing a song. This helps with your breathing and channels nervous energy.
2. Wash your face and hands with a very hot washcloth.
3. Cup your hands under warm running water. Let it fill your hands and pour out.
4. Hug a partner, spouse, child, or friend.
5. Pet a cat or dog.
6. Hold your hands open, palms facing up, and focus on breathing slowly.
7. Run your hands along something with texture, such as fake fur or textured carpeting. Focus on your hands and what they're feeling.
8. Drum your hands on a soft but resistant surface, such as a mattress.
9. Place your hands flat against the wall and push against it, as if you're holding the wall up.
10. Focus on your senses. What are you hearing? What are you seeing? What are you smelling? What are you touching?

Many of us are great procrastinators, living by the motto "Why do today what I can put off until tomorrow?" Would you consider yourself a procrastinator? If so, you can't afford to put off reading this section.

Putting work, projects, or tasks off almost always has negative consequences, one of which is disturbed sleep. Getting your work done can be seen as another way of managing your stress. You can choose to put your time and energy into accomplishing what is before you and reap the benefits or put it off and worry about it. Tasks left undone can even intrude into your dreams at night and, in extreme cases, lead to nightmares.

Avoiding procrastination takes some discipline. There are certain techniques, however, that can help:

• **MAKE A "TO-DO" LIST FOR THE DAY,** then rank your list from most to least important. Start with the most important and work your way through them, checking each off as you complete it. If unexpected circumstances limit what you can accomplish that day, you will have put your limited time and energy toward the most important tasks. And this will leave you with a sense of accomplishment.

• **FINISH WHAT YOU START.** Leaving projects half-done is sometimes worse than not starting them at all. An incomplete job will occupy your mind and make relaxing difficult. Also, work that is partly done robs you of the satisfaction that comes with closure.

• **KEEP PROMISES TO DO TASKS ON TIME.** Make schedules and stick with them. When promised work is late, it only becomes more difficult to face as time goes by.

• **LEARN TO SAY "NO."** Sometimes we procrastinate because we feel overwhelmed by all of our commitments. Still, we continue to volunteer for tasks or projects because we don't want to tell someone "no." To combat this habit, make an effort to look realistically at your schedule and responsibilities before you commit to optional activities, and realize that knowing when to say "no" is better for your sleep and your health than worrying about tasks you can't hope to accomplish.

With some planning and a little self-discipline, you may find it easier to relax at night.

TIRED OR BORED?

Have you ever had to fight to keep your eyes open during a meeting or battled the head-nods while listening to a presentation? You probably attributed your desire to doze to the boring nature of the activity. But consider this: Children—who tend to get the amount of sleep their bodies need—don't get sleepy when faced with a boring situation; they get restless. So if sitting through a "sleeper of a speech" has you fighting to stay awake, consider it a hint from your body that you are not getting the sleep you need. This is especially vital when you are driving long distances. If you feel you have to turn up the radio or open a window just to stay awake during a "boring" drive, you are most likely too tired to be driving. The solution is not distraction but sleep.

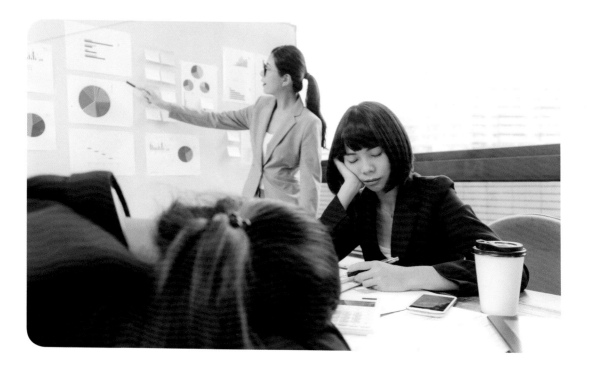

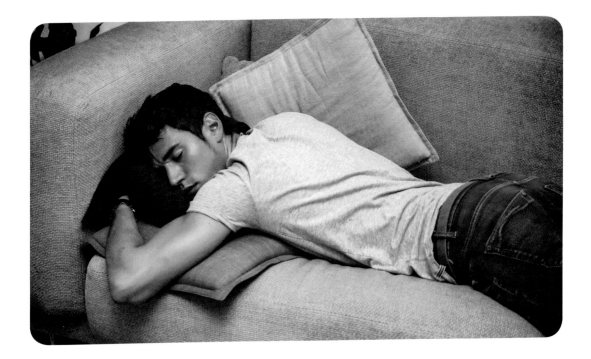

NAP SPARINGLY

Some people swear by naps; others find that napping during the day disrupts their sleep at night. Naps can be beneficial or detrimental, depending on how we use them. The urge to nap is greatest about eight hours after we awaken from a night's sleep. This is when our body temperature begins the first of two daily dips (the other, more dramatic dip, which we discussed earlier in this chapter, occurs at night). A short nap in the early to midafternoon can bring a renewed sense of energy and alertness. A nap in the late afternoon or early evening, on the other hand, can disrupt your sleep cycle and make it difficult to fall asleep when you retire for the night.

To benefit most from a nap, take it no later than midafternoon and keep it under 30 minutes. If you nap for a longer period, your body lapses into a deeper phase of sleep, which can leave you feeling groggy when you awaken. If you are severely sleep-deprived and can't go on without a nap, it is better to sleep for a longer time to allow yourself to go through one complete sleep cycle. An average sleep cycle takes about 90 minutes in most people.

If you find you need a nap every day, take it at the same time so your body can develop a rhythm that incorporates the nap. If you try to take a nap but are unable to sleep, simply resting with your eyes closed may help restore some alertness and energy.

It's also possible to use naps to temper the negative effects of an anticipated sleep deficit. For instance, if you know you are going to be up late because of special plans, take a prolonged nap of two to three hours earlier in the day. This has been shown to reduce fatigue at the normal bedtime and improve alertness, although it may throw off your normal sleep rhythm temporarily.

NAPPING TIPS

• **Keep naps short.** Aim to nap for only 10–30 minutes. The longer you nap, the more likely you are to feel groggy afterward.

• **The best time for a nap is usually midafternoon,** around 2 or 3 p.m. This is when you might experience post-lunch sleepiness or a lower level of alertness. Naps taken during this time are also less likely to interfere with nighttime sleep.

• **Create a restful environment.** Nap in a quiet, dark place with a comfortable room temperature and few distractions.

• **After napping, be sure to give yourself time** to wake up before resuming activities—particularly those that require a quick or sharp response.

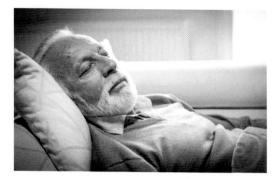

EAT AND DRINK WISELY

How much of a direct effect diet has on sleep is still unclear. It's safe to say, though, that a balanced, varied diet full of fresh fruits, vegetables, whole grains, and low-fat protein sources can help your body function optimally and help ward off chronic conditions such as heart disease. Controlling portion sizes so you're taking in only enough calories to maintain a healthy weight can help keep diseases such as diabetes at bay. And since chronic diseases and the drugs required to treat them can interfere with sleep, eating wisely can help you safeguard your health and your sleep.

Adjusting your eating routine may also help you get a better night's sleep. Most Americans eat a light breakfast, a moderate lunch, and a large meal in the evening. Yet leaving the largest meal to the end of the day may not be the best choice, since it can result in uncomfortable distension and possibly heartburn when you retire for the night. You might want to try reversing that pattern for a more sleep-friendly meal plan:

• Eat a substantial breakfast. Because you are breaking your nighttime fast and consuming the nutrients you will need for energy throughout the morning, breakfast should be your largest meal of the day. Whole-grain breads and cereals, yogurt, and fruit are just a few examples of good breakfast choices.

• Opt for a moderate lunch. Choose brown rice, pasta, or whole-grain bread and a serving of protein—fish, eggs, chicken, meat, or beans.

• Finish with a light dinner. It is particularly important to eat lightly for your evening meal in order to prepare for a good night's sleep. Plan to finish your meal at least two hours before going to bed, preferably longer.

If you need a little something to eat before you hit the sack, you'll find suggestions for late-night snacks a bit later in this chapter.

In addition, you may want to try these tips:

• Reduce or eliminate caffeine, especially in the late afternoon and evening. Ideally you want to avoid caffeine within six hours of bedtime. Caffeine is a stimulant, which is why so many of us reach for that cup of coffee in the morning to get us going. And it's true that some individuals can drink caffeinated beverages all day long and still sleep soundly at night. But if you're having trouble sleeping, then limiting your caffeine intake should be one of the first steps you try to help improve your sleep. Be aware that coffee is not the only source of caffeine. Many sodas and teas, chocolate, and some medications, especially those for headaches, also contain caffeine. Check labels to help eliminate such sources of stimulation.

• Some people are sensitive to the flavor enhancer and preservative monosodium glutamate (MSG). In susceptible individuals, it can cause digestive upset, headaches, and other reactions that can interfere with sleep. MSG is found in some processed foods and in some Asian foods. Try avoiding foods that contain MSG to see if it helps you sleep better.

• Drink the majority of your fluids for the day by the end of dinner. A full bladder may be cutting into your sleep time. Drink plenty of water throughout the day. Water is essential to healthy bodily functions. Shoot for eight glasses, or two quarts, per day. But be sure to drink the majority of your fluids before dinnertime so you won't be making numerous trips to the bathroom during your sleeping hours.

• Skip the alcohol. Despite making you feel drowsy, alcohol may actually be disturbing your sleep. Avoid drinking alcohol within two hours of bedtime.

SCHEDULE YOUR SLEEP

It might seem unnatural to schedule your sleep like you would an important appointment, but this is one of the most vital principles to getting a good night's rest. Here are several ideas for keeping a scheduled sleep routine.

ESTABLISH A BEDTIME RITUAL

Most of us begin our day with a morning routine. It helps us prepare ourselves physically and mentally for the day. So why not establish a bedtime routine that helps to prepare you for sleep? The purpose of a bedtime ritual is to send a signal to your body and mind that it's time to sleep.

You probably already have some regular bedtime habits, even if you haven't realized it. Brushing and flossing your teeth, lowering the thermostat, and setting your alarm clock may all be part of your evening routine. To help you get to sleep, you should perform these activities in the same manner and order every night.

Avoid activities that are stimulating or laden with emotion right before bedtime. Starting to assemble your

 WHAT'S YOUR RITUAL?

A bedtime ritual can be anything you want it to be as long as you do it each night. An appealing ritual for many might include: a light snack, laying clothes out for the next day, a warm bath or shower, brushing teeth, listening to soft music and/or reading, followed by lights out. Begin your ritual 30 to 60 minutes before your bedtime, and don't rush through it.

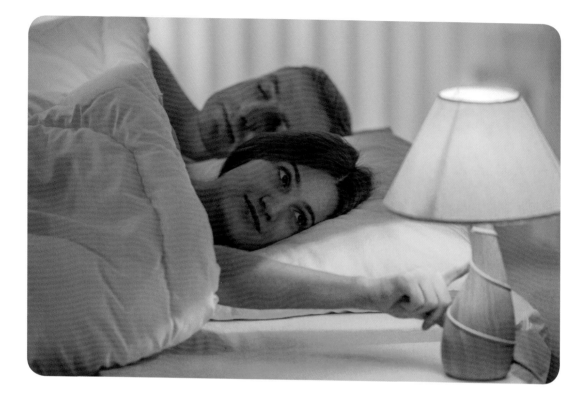

child's new playhouse or paying a stack of bills 30 minutes before bed would not be wise. Begin those types of activities earlier in the evening, and end them in time to go unhurriedly through your bedtime routine.

Establishing some type of bedtime ritual also provides closure to your day and allows you to go to bed and sleep with a more quiet body and mind.

Make a standing appointment with your pillow. It's often too easy to put off bedtime to do one more chore, watch one more episode, or read one more page. So try writing or typing "bedtime" into the same time slot of your planner or calendar every day. It might seem a bit silly at first, but seeing your bedtime written down—just like your other appointments—may help reinforce its importance. Having a set end-time to your day clearly noted in your calendar may also help you avoid overscheduling or planning activities too late in the evening.

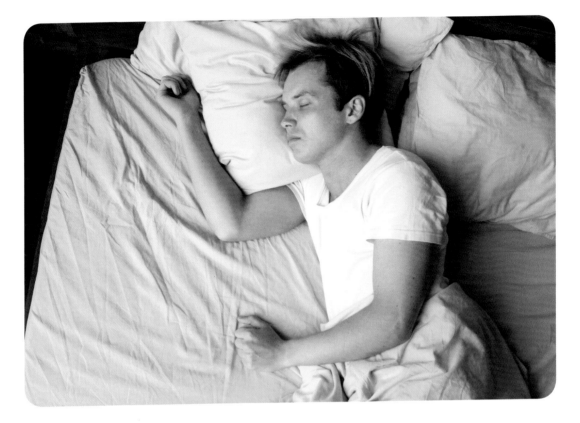

STAY REGULAR

Some people think going to bed on a schedule is only for children. While it's good for children to have a regular bedtime, it's also very good for adults who want to sleep like children when they hit the sack.

The idea is to go to bed and wake up at the same time each day, even on weekends. If you feel you must get up later on weekends, allow yourself a maximum of one hour later arising. This regularity helps set your internal sleep-wake clock. Within weeks of keeping a regular sleep-wake schedule, you will begin to feel more alert than if you were keeping a variable sleep-wake routine. Not only will a stable rhythm of sleeping and waking improve the quality of your sleep, but it will probably also improve the quality of your life. Try it for six weeks and see the difference it makes in your energy and alertness.

EARLY TO BED

There is nothing childish or old-fashioned about going to bed early. Listen to what your body is telling you. If you find yourself yawning at 9 p.m., go to bed. If you resist this urge even by 30 minutes you might miss the window in your sleep-wake cycle that could have put you into a deep sleep faster. Don't want to miss a favorite show? Use your DVR.

Chapter 3: Ease Into Sleep

NOW THAT YOU KNOW HOW to prepare for sleep during the day and schedule it at night, you're ready for bed. But before you peel those sheets back, consider how you might prepare your body and mind for that relaxing and peaceful sleep for which you long. The hour before bedtime is the most critical for good sleep. When used properly, the time right before bed can help you let go of the stressful, anxiety-provoking events of the day and promote a restful night's sleep. But if that last hour before slumber is not used properly, it can set the stage for a long night of tossing and turning. Try some of the following ideas to see which work best for you.

ESTABLISH A BEDTIME RITUAL

As discussed in chapter 2, establishing a bedtime ritual helps prepare you mentally and physically for sleep. Repeating the same activities before bed each night will signal your body and mind that it's time to wind down and sleep. You probably already have some regular bedtime habits, such as locking the doors, lowering the thermostat, brushing your teeth, and setting your alarm clock. The key to turning them into a sleep-encouraging ritual is to perform them in the same manner and order every night. Begin your ritual 30 to 60 minutes prior to crawling into bed. And avoid potentially stimulating or stressful activities, such as browsing social media posts or answering work e-mails, during your bedtime ritual.

SEEK SERENITY

The key to preparing for sleep is to establish an atmosphere of peace and calm. Ease your mind and body with quiet yet pleasurable activities. You will create a sense of inner well-being that allows sleep to come quickly and easily. Most people find one of the following works well for them. Experiment with several if you're not sure.

- **Read to relax.** But choose your reading material with care. The idea is to read something light that won't stimulate your mind. In other words, you probably don't want to crack that new crime thriller. Better choices would be a popular magazine, a short story, or perhaps devotional reading.

- **Listen to music.** Choose music that relaxes you. In general, soft instrumental music has the most calming effect. Hard driving rock and pop beats often pull you into the music, causing you to be more awake, especially if the tunes are familiar. Another sound alternative might be playing a CD or mp3 of nature sounds.

- **Try meditation or prayer.** These activities, which help many people relax, can also help you be at peace with whatever is on your mind. More information about meditation can be found in chapter 8.

- **Watch television, but only if it helps you relax.** Watching television is fine if you use some discipline. Falling asleep with the TV on in your bedroom is not the best way to start your sleep. In most cases, you have to awaken to turn it off, which forces you to have to fall asleep again. The idea is to stay asleep once you doze off. A better use of television is to watch it earlier in the evening and practice other relaxation techniques right before bed. If you must watch right before bed, don't watch in your bedroom.

TAKE A WARM BATH

One popular way to relax the body and slow down the mind is a warm bath, and you may find it fits the bill for you. But you may want to do some experimenting with your timing. Some people find a nice hot bath just before bed makes them drowsy and ready to drop into sleep. If you do, enjoy. On the other hand, some people find that a hot bath is actually stimulating or that it makes them too uncomfortably warm when they slip into bed. If you find a just-before-bed bath makes it harder for you to fall asleep, consider taking the bath earlier, a couple of hours before bed. An earlier bath may enhance the gradual drop in body temperature that normally occurs at night and help trigger drowsiness.

RECIPE FOR A SOOTHING BATH

Consider making your bath more relaxing by:

• Dimming the lights and/or using candles to create a calming atmosphere

• Playing soft music in the background

• Reading pleasurable material that you find relaxing

• Adding 2 cups of Epsom salts to the bathwater to ease sore or tired muscles

• Laying back and using a towel or waterproof pillow to support your head

PRACTICE RELAXATION TECHNIQUES

An excellent way to quiet your body and mind before bedtime is to use active relaxation techniques such as progressive muscle relaxation, abdominal breathing, and visualization. These techniques help you to deliberately clear your mind of intrusive thoughts, wring the tension from your body, and put yourself into a peaceful state.

PROGRESSIVE MUSCLE RELAXATION (PMR)

When you tense a muscle for a few seconds, it naturally wants to relax. That is how PMR works. You start at your toes and deliberately tense one muscle group at a time, progressively working your way up the body. To prepare, lie on your back on the floor or on a couch or recliner in a room other than your bedroom. Begin by scrunching your toes as hard as you can for ten seconds, while keeping the rest of your body relaxed. Then relax your toes, and tighten and release your calf muscles, again leaving your other muscles relaxed. Then move on to your thigh muscles. Continue through the muscle groups of the buttocks, abdomen, chest,

forearms, shoulders, neck, and face. Take your time at it; performing the muscle relaxation from toes to head one time should take at least 20 minutes. By the time you work your way through the muscle groups, you should feel very relaxed. If you don't, repeat the entire cycle one more time.

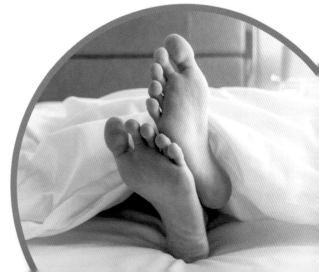

ABDOMINAL BREATHING

Rhythmic breathing is one of the best ways to help your body relax. There are many variations. This particular technique appears simple, but you'll need a little practice to do it properly. First, lie down on your back and begin to breathe normally. Now place your hand on your lower abdomen, just at your belt line, and slowly fill your lungs with air to the point that you can feel this portion of your abdomen rise. Take in as much air as you can and hold it for a couple of seconds. Then slowly release all the air in your lungs. Try to pay attention to nothing but the slow intake and release of air, the rhythmic rising and falling of your abdomen; don't rush. Repeat this eight to ten times.

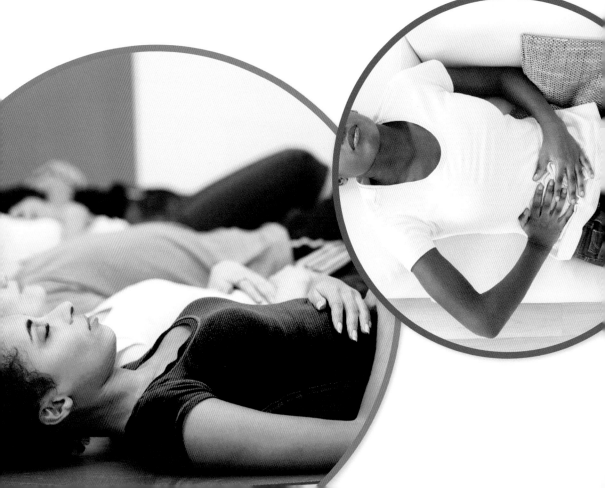

VISUALIZATION

Imagine your favorite vacation spot. Maybe it's sitting on the sand with your bare feet being massaged by the ocean surf, or scuba diving off some coral reef. Alternately, think of an activity you find especially relaxing: drawing, cooking, hiking, walking your dog, even shopping. The idea behind visualization is to use your imagination to envision something that tells your mind to enjoy itself instead of being focused on some worry or concern. It can be anything you find soothing. As you lie in bed, close your eyes and literally "go" to that place or "do" that activity in your mind. Chances are good that you will be sleeping peacefully in short order.

SNACK LIGHTLY BEFORE BED

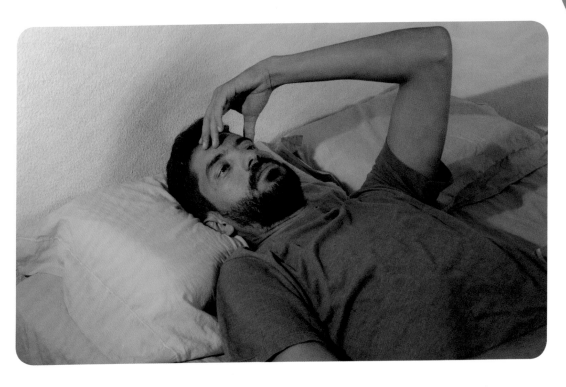

There's nothing like a grumbling stomach to keep you awake. So if hunger pangs strike as you're preparing for bed, have a light snack. Research indicates that a light snack can help you sleep more soundly. The emphasis, of course, is on light. Bedtime is no time to stuff yourself. An overly full belly can be just as detrimental to sleep as an empty one.

There are various theories about what you should have as a snack before bed. One age-old suggestion is warm milk. Some research has suggested that milk might be helpful because it contains tryptophan, a naturally occurring amino acid that the body uses to make serotonin; serotonin is a brain chemical that has a calming, sleep-promoting effect. Tryptophan is also found in a variety of other foods, such as turkey, tuna, peanuts, and cheese.

Other researchers emphasize the importance of eating a nighttime snack that is high in carbohydrates, such as bread, potatoes, cereal, or juice. The carbohydrates, they contend, help usher tryptophan into the brain, where it is converted into serotonin.

Some sleep scientists recommend eating foods that are rich in magnesium and/or calcium. These minerals have a calming effect on the nervous system, and even a slight deficiency of them, they say, can affect sleep. Dairy foods are good sources of calcium. Sources of magnesium include fruits such as apples, apricots, avocados, bananas, and peaches; nuts; and whole-grain breads and cereals.

You might want to experiment with snacks from these various groups to see if they help you sleep. There's no guarantee they'll lead you to a good night's sleep, but you may find some of them helpful.

When choosing a snack before bed, another important point is that you should avoid foods that may promote heartburn, indigestion, gas, or other upsets. That means you should probably avoid greasy, fatty, and spicy foods. If you're lactose intolerant, skip the warm milk—or use a lactose-free variety. And if MSG causes you problems, don't treat yourself to those Chinese takeout leftovers.

HAVE SOME WARM MILK

The sleep-inducing properties of warm milk are legendary. Zap a microwaveable mug of fresh milk on high for 1 minute; stir and test temperature before drinking. Or, heat the milk in a small saucepan over low heat until it's warm but not boiling. Drink before going to bed.

DON'T GO TO BED ANGRY

You've just gotten off the phone with a relative who infuriates you every time you talk with them. Every single time they call, they launch into all the things they see wrong with the way you're living your life. Flying into your bedroom like a whirlwind, you try to get ready for bed. You're burning with anger. You lie down on the bed and repeatedly slam your fist into your pillow as you try to find a comfortable position. But you can't fall asleep...you're on fire.

Too often people go to bed when their mind is a raging fury, agonizing over some event of the day. Don't make this mistake. You don't want your bed to be a place for anger or worry. Your bedroom should produce a feeling of peace and contentment.

When your emotions have boiled over, stay out of the bed and the bedroom until you cool down. Try journaling or writing your frustrations down on paper to help unburden your mind. Or try one of the relaxation techniques described in this chapter (pages 57–59) to unwind your tangled emotions. Once you've calmed down, then you can retreat to bed.

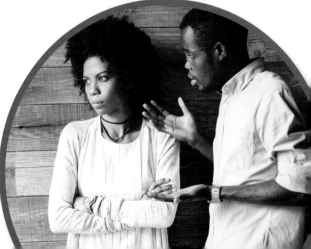

SKIP THE TIMER

If you're one of those folks who sets the timer on the television, radio, or the audiobook on your smartphone and drifts off listening to it, you might want to break yourself of the habit. Without realizing it, you may actually fight off sleep just to hear the end of that episode or the last bars of a favorite song. And if you condition yourself to fall asleep only when you have that background noise, you may not be able to fall back to sleep without it when you wake up in the middle of the night. So you either struggle to fall back asleep without it or wake yourself up just to turn the device back on—neither of which is likely to improve your sleep overall.

STOP TRYING

While lying in bed, tossing and turning, you may become frustrated at your inability to slip into slumber, perhaps even repeating over and over, "I've got to go to sleep." The more you try to will yourself into sleep, the more conscious you become of not being able to doze off.

But sleep is unlike most activities in life. While trying harder is often the surest path to success in business, sports, or other waking activities, it is the surest path to failure when you want to sleep. Attempting to force yourself to sleep simply won't work. It only increases anxiety and tension. Sleep is most easily achieved in an atmosphere of total relaxation. Your mind should be empty of thought or turned to soothing and calming thoughts. Your body should be relaxed, your muscles free of tension.

GET UP

If you find you can't fall asleep, the best solution is to get out of bed. That's right. Contrary to popular belief, the solution is not to stay in bed. If this happens with any frequency, and you do stay in bed, you may begin to associate your room and bed with feeling frustrated, uncomfortable, and unhappy. When you walk into your room, you'll immediately begin to worry about how long it will take to fall asleep. Consequently, it will take longer to drift off into slumber.

Let your body associate any feelings of wakefulness with some other part of your home. Go to the kitchen for a drink of water. Go into another room and read, knit, draw. Almost any activity will do as long as it's calming, relaxing, and doesn't require intense concentration. Gradually, you'll become tired and bored. Usually, within 15 to 20 minutes, your body will be ready for you to try to sleep again.

Once you begin to feel drowsy, return to your bedroom and bed to sleep. If you still can't fall asleep within a brief time (about ten minutes), get up again and engage in some quiet activity in another room. Repeat this process as often as it is necessary throughout the night. Use this same procedure if you awaken in the middle of the night and do not fall back to sleep within about ten minutes.

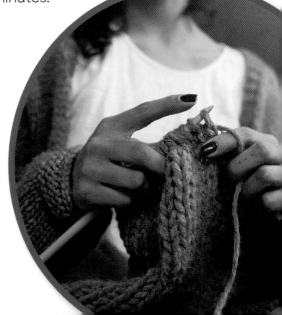

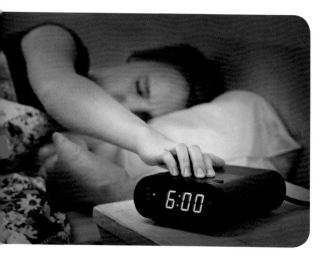

HIDE THE ALARM CLOCK

The bedside clock can be your number one enemy when you're having difficulty falling asleep. It acts as a constant reminder of how long it is taking you to fall to sleep and how little time you have left before needing to get up. It wakes you up just looking at it. So rather than letting it stare you in the face all night, set it for the waking time desired, then move it out of your line of sight (but not out of earshot) or turn it to face away from you.

DOES COUNTING SHEEP WORK?

The oldest trick in the book may not be such a great trick after all. It was considered a given that the repetitive, monotonous activity of counting sheep would bore you to sleep. But a group of researchers at Oxford University decided to test that age-old theory. According to their results, counting sheep is actually so boring that it doesn't keep your attention long enough for you to relax your body and mind for sleep. What did seem to help the insomniacs to fall asleep an average of more than 20 minutes sooner was visualizing a relaxing, inviting scene. Check out our discussion of visualization on page 59 to learn more about this sleep-promoting technique.

Chapter 4: Control Your Sleep Environment

SOME PEOPLE CAN FALL TO sleep anywhere. For most of us, though, our sleep environment has a substantial, if often overlooked, effect on our ability to get a good night's sleep. So let's take a look at how you can make your sleep environment more conducive to restful slumber.

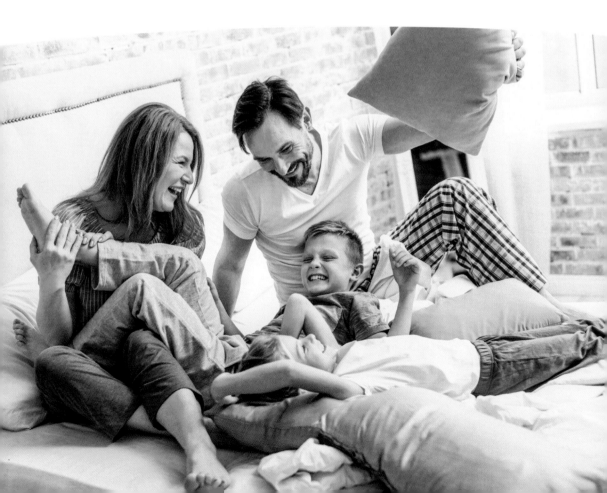

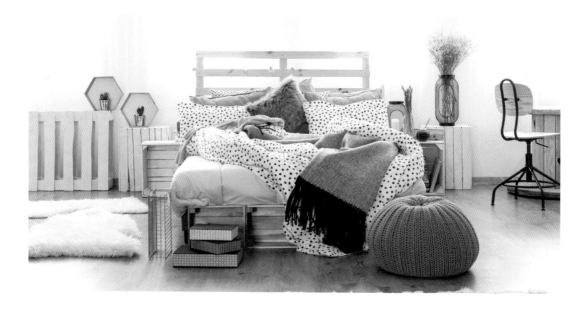

MAKE YOUR BED A HAVEN

Most of us think of our bed as a place to sleep. But many people also use their bed for watching television, listening to the radio, talking on the phone, texting, answering e-mails, eating, reading, or playing games. If you really want to sleep better, however, you shouldn't do any of these nonsleep activities in bed. When you do, the bed and bedroom can become associated with these activities rather than with sleep. Instead, you want to condition your mind and body to become drowsy and ready for sleep when you get into your bed, not ready and alert for a chat with a friend or a drama on TV.

Some people even go so far as to do work in bed. While this practice may help you catch up on paperwork, it can seriously disrupt your sleep. When you do work in bed, all of the associated stress becomes related to the bed and bedroom. Just getting into bed at night may subsequently cause your heart rate to increase, your muscles to tighten, and your thoughts to race. Whether you consciously realize it, the sheets, blankets, and pillows can become associated with your work. Their very sight and smell may cause thoughts of work to flood your mind as you try to fall asleep.

The single exception to the rule about banning nonsleep activities in bed may be sex. We say "may be," because it depends on the effect that sex has on you and your bed partner. For some people, sexual activity is very relaxing and tiring and tends to make them sleepy. If that's the case for both partners, then having sex before sleep may be just the ticket for a restful night. However, some people find sexual activity actually refreshes and energizes them, making them more alert. And, for some folks, relationship problems, frustrations, or negative feelings about sex can make it far from pleasant or relaxing. For couples in which either partner finds sexual activity too stimulating or too fraught with negative emotions to be conducive to sleep, sex might best be left for another time and even a different room. It's important for couples to talk and determine what works best for both partners in terms of helping or harming their efforts at getting a good night's sleep.

CLEAR BEDROOM CLUTTER

Is your bedroom a sanctuary that feels calm, looks clean, and invites you to relax? Or is it strewn with clothes and accessories, shoes, magazines, books, and/or work files? To transform your bedroom into a restful, welcoming sleep chamber, start by cleaning. If your bedroom has been doubling as an office, move your computer, briefcase, and related stuff to another location or hide it all behind a folding screen. Pitch or relocate items that might distract you from sleep. Pare down knickknacks, excess furniture, and other clutter that does nothing but collect dust. Then add subtle artwork, bedding, wall coverings, and window treatments that you find soothing.

CHOOSE THE RIGHT MATTRESS

We spend about one-third of our lives asleep, and most of this time is spent on a mattress. Despite the amount of time we spend in bed, many of us ignore our mattress until the springs start poking us through the mattress pad. But a mattress has a lot to do with the quality of sleep and, therefore, with how we feel during the day. So give some thought and attention to the type of mattress you use to ensure a good night's sleep and a well-rested feeling the following day.

When selecting a mattress, you need to make decisions about:

- Firmness
- Type of mattress and bed
- Size

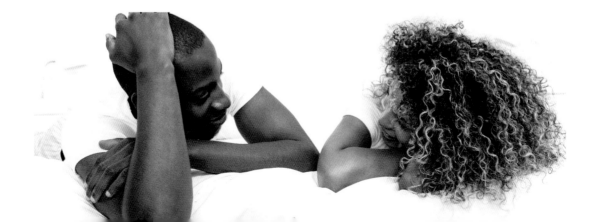

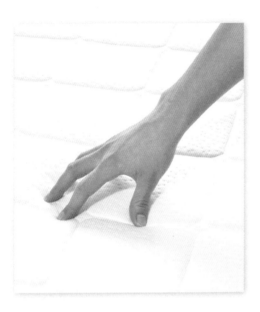

DON'T FORGET THE CUSHIONING

The top layers of mattress cushioning are often what sell the customer. Comfort is what most people look for. But consider what the padding is made of. A cotton-polyester blend on top of polyurethane foam doesn't breathe well, yet this is the material used in many mattresses. Wool is a better material for layers closest to your body. Wool whisks moisture away from your body and keeps you dry while you sleep.

MATTRESS FIRMNESS

Don't assume soft and fluffy is best. Poor support can lead to muscle stiffness as well as neck and back pain. Make sure your mattress isn't too soft and doesn't contain bumps, valleys, or depressions. Of course, too stiff isn't great, either. A mattress that is too hard can put pressure on the shoulders and hips. The ideal surface is gently supportive and firm, not rock hard or squishy. The mattress should mold to your body while supporting it.

Keep in mind that mattresses don't last forever. Gradually, over time, they lose their firmness and support. The average life of a mattress is ten years, although most people keep them much longer. Once your mattress has developed lumps and sags, it is definitely time to replace it.

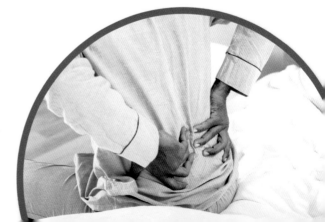

MATTRESS TYPES

Mattresses come in different types. What are your options?

• *Polyurethane foam mattresses.* These come in different degrees of firmness but often make people hot while sleeping. As you sleep, your body loses a pint or more of moisture per night. When a mattress doesn't "breathe" well or allow air to circulate, it can make you feel hot and sweaty.

• *Innerspring mattresses.* These mattresses consist of rows of tempered steel coils layered between insulation and padding. Firmness and durability is based on the thickness of the wire and the number of coils. The higher the coil count, the firmer the mattress.

• *Waterbeds.* Waterbeds don't breathe, and they tend to sag under your body's heaviest parts. Some people love waterbeds and wouldn't sleep on anything else. But before you buy one, sleep on someone else's to see if it meets your expectations.

Most people choose innerspring mattresses because they offer many options for firmness, are cooler and drier because the air circulates around the coils, and are widely available.

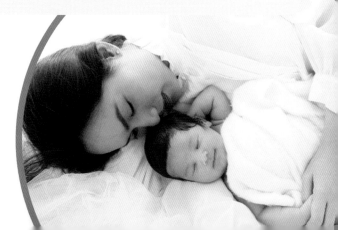

MATTRESS SIZE

Along with deciding what kind of mattress you want, you need to figure out what size. As a rule, bigger is better. You don't want to fight for space every night or get kicked, elbowed, or shoved on a regular basis. A healthy sleeper moves around from 15 to 30 times during the night, and cramped conditions can make sleeping awkward, uncomfortable, and altogether frustrating. Indeed, some decades-old research suggests that sleeping in the same bed as someone else is less restful than sleeping alone. Also, as you and your bed partner get older, your sleep will become more restless and you may require extra room in bed. So, you can either consider sleeping in separate beds or get the largest mattress that fits in your bedroom and your budget. You might also want to try one of the newer mattresses that, according to their manufacturers, are designed to minimize the movement and disruption one bed partner feels when the other tosses, turns, and gets in and out of bed.

Regardless of which mattress or bed you buy, always try it out in the store before making it yours. Salespeople expect you to lie on their beds as part of your decision-making process. Assume your normal sleeping position, and stay there for a while to determine how it feels. If you have a bed partner, have them join you on the mattress. Even better, ask if the mattress comes with a trial period that allows you to exchange or return it if it's not right for you. And remember: Be picky—you'll be spending a lot of your life on that mattress.

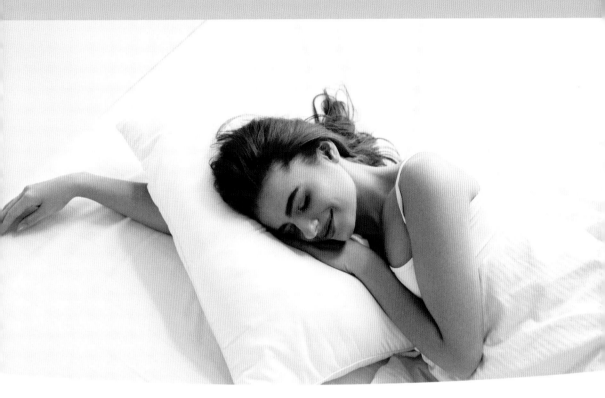

PICK YOUR PILLOW WISELY

Like the choice of a mattress, the choice of a pillow is a very personal matter. Although some people can sleep with their head on a block of wood, most of us are very particular about the type of pillow we use. Your head weighs more than ten pounds, so your pillow needs to provide you with support as well as comfort.

A good pillow supports you in just the right places. It should keep your head in line with your back and spine. But different sleeping positions require different pillows. If you tend to sleep on your side, you need a firm pillow that supports your head and neck. If you prefer sleeping on your back, a medium to firm pillow will offer you more cushion. Those who sleep on their stomach should choose a soft pillow to ease strain on the neck.

Most pillows are made with synthetic fibers or foam, which are more friendly to allergy-prone people

TEST YOUR PILLOW

If you're trying to determine whether your pillow is ready for replacement, try these tests. If you own a polyester pillow, fold it in half and place a shoe on top. If the pillow unfolds and knocks the shoe off, it is still good. If the shoe wins, the pillow probably needs replacing. If you have a feather pillow, fold it in half and squeeze out as much air as you can. (Leave the shoe out of this contest.) When you release the pillow, it should unfold on its own. If not, its goose is cooked and the pillow needs to be replaced.

and easy to wash. If you must have a down or feather pillow, make sure it doesn't cause an allergic reaction in your sleep partner before you purchase it.

Other types of pillows include orthopedic varieties that are designed to relieve pain and stiffness in the neck or back. Orthopedic pillows are more expensive than conventional pillows, but medical insurance may cover their purchase if your doctor prescribes them. You can purchase these pillows at a surgical supply store.

Also available are pillows designed to reduce or eliminate snoring. Despite the rather optimistic claims about these pillows, they are rarely effective. It's better to address the snoring problem directly with your doctor rather than muffle it with a futile search for the perfect pillow.

Most important, find a pillow that makes you feel comfortable. And when your pillow starts to lose its shape or support, it's time to get a new one. Experiment with a variety of types, and stick with the one that provides you with the best night's sleep.

HUMIDIFY YOUR HOME

You're hot, and your throat is parched. Each swallow is agonizingly difficult. Your skin is dry and cracked, and your eyes are burning. All you can think of is a tall, cool glass of water. Where are you? The Sahara? Death Valley? The planet Venus? No, you're in bed in the typical North American home in winter, where the artificial heat that keeps us warm also dries out the air we breathe.

Although most of us prefer a temperature of 68 degrees or higher in the winter, we may pay a price for all that warmth. While heating systems warm our surroundings, they also remove a lot of moisture from the air. As you breathe this hot, dry air, water is also removed from your breathing passages, which can lead to throat or nasal discomfort or even upper airway infection. (Influenza viruses thrive in an atmosphere of low humidity.) If you ever feel the urge for a glass of water in the middle of the night to soothe a dry, parched throat, especially during the winter months, chances are good that dry air is a factor.

Fortunately, there is a relatively simple solution to the dry air caused by indoor heating: a humidifier. A humidifier adds moisture to the air, makes sleep easier, and provides a more comfortable and healthful environment. Humidifying your home can also ease some of your discomfort if you have a respiratory infection. If you can't afford a whole-house humidifier, get a portable room humidifier and keep it in the bedroom. Just be sure to follow the manufacturer's cleaning and filter-replacement guidelines to combat the growth of bacteria and mold.

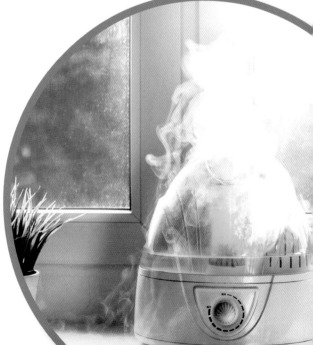

CONTROL THE TEMPERATURE

Sleep experts say a cool bedroom between 60 and 67 degrees Fahrenheit makes for the best sleep. Our body temperature naturally dips to initiate sleep and a cooler bedroom can help facilitate this. In addition to a cooler room temperature, try wearing socks to bed. Keeping your extremities warm helps dilate your blood vessels so they can better redistribute heat throughout your body. For babies and toddlers, the best room temperature for sleeping is between 65 and 70 degrees Fahrenheit.

MINIMIZE DISTRACTIONS

Your bedroom should be a sanctuary free from all potential sleep distractions. Remove electronic devices such as televisions, computers, laptops, tablets, cell phones, e-readers, and video games from your bedroom. If you must use these devices in your bedroom, use them from a desk or chair rather than from your bed. Your body needs to know that the bed is only for sleep and sex.

LIMIT THE LIGHT

Light tells your body it's time to wake up, so the darker your bedroom, the better. If an outdoor light shines into your room at night, purchase shades or curtains to block it out. If necessary, use a night-light for nighttime bathroom trips, but keep it away from your immediate sleeping area. If you aren't able to sufficiently keep light out of your bedroom during sleep hours, purchase eye shades; they're available at most drugstores as well as through websites and catalogs that sell accessories for travelers.

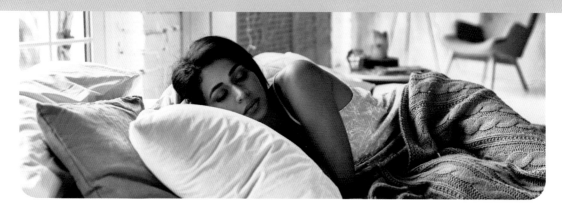

WHITE-OUT THE NOISE

Our sleeping environment is rarely sound-free. It may be plagued by a snoring bedmate, barking dogs, the roar of planes overhead, the neighbor's loud music, or even the incessant early-morning chirping of birds. The best solution, of course, is to eliminate the noise, but that's often easier said than done. So instead of trying to eliminate all nighttime noise pollution, try masking the noise with a white-noise machine.

White-noise machines are sound-producing devices. With the push of a button, a white-noise machine makes a soft, whooshing noise that can drown out many of the sudden and unpredictable noises that can disturb sleep. The white noise is easy to get used to and is actually quite soothing. More sophisticated models can produce the sounds of rain, wind, waves, or other nature sounds, although these may be too stimulating or distracting for some folks.

Unlike the television or a radio, the noise produced by a white-noise machine or app does not tend to awaken you from sleep because the volume is constant and the sound itself is unchanging. White-noise machines range in price and are available from specialty shops and websites, mail-order catalogs, and even some department stores.

In addition to white-noise machines, there are also apps that can play white noise from your smartphone. Just make sure that having your phone nearby while trying to sleep doesn't provide a tempting distraction.

PLUG YOUR EARS

Earplugs are another option for dealing with the annoying environmental noise that can make it difficult to fall asleep or startle you awake just as you drift off. Soft, sound-muffling earplugs are available in a variety of materials at most drugstores.

You can also purchase noise-cancelling or noise-isolating headphones that can deliver white noise directly to your ears while minimizing the outside noise that gets in.

GIVE PETS THE BOOT

Many of us let our pet(s) sleep in bed with us. While this sleeping situation can be comforting to both human and pet, it can also disrupt sleep.

Some pets like to nuzzle up during the night. As you move, they move with you. By morning, you may find that you have been herded onto a tiny patch of the mattress while your pet has sprawled out freely on the rest. And, like people, pets change position various times throughout the night, which can awaken you. Add another person to the bed along with a pet or two and you have enough movement to simulate eight hours of earthquake aftershocks.

Then there are pets that wake their owners just for company. (Ever awoken to find one of your pet's favorite toys on your pillow?) If any of these scenarios sound familiar, it's time to bar your pet from your bed. If you must, keep the door to your bedroom closed when you sleep to keep your pet from wandering in. You might at first feel bad about banning your furry friend, but rest assured your pet will not love you less, and you'll both sleep better in the end.

SLEEPING AWAY FROM HOME

Even in the lavish surroundings of a four-star hotel, you usually don't sleep as well as you do in your own bed. The poor sleep that often occurs in a strange environment is known as the first-night effect. This name is appropriate because sleep often improves considerably after as little as one night away from home. One trick to getting sound sleep when away from home is to make the environment seem more familiar and homelike. A simple way to do this is to bring along some objects from home. Bring your own pillow, pictures of family, or other reminders of your own bedroom and home. Also try to follow your usual routine in the hour before bed. If you read before bed, bring along a book or grab the local newspaper. If you usually take a shower, do the same. Give your body all its usual clues that bedtime is approaching.

If, on the other hand, you find you sleep better away from home, try to determine why. What did the new sleep environment have that your bedroom at home does not? No pets? Better pillows? A firmer mattress? A quieter environment? Distance from life's problems? When you get home, try some of our suggestions for making your sleep environment more sleep-friendly.

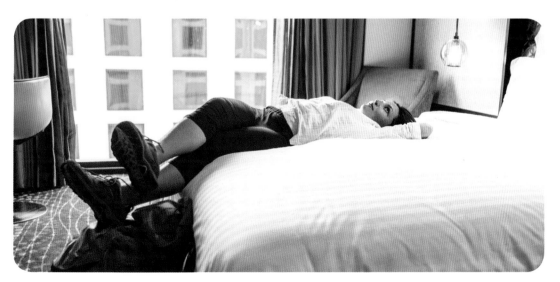

MOVING? CHECK OUT THE NEIGHBORHOOD

If you're planning on moving, check out prospective new homes and neighborhoods for noise pollution before you sign a deal. Here are some tips to help you screen out sleep-stealing housing situations.

• Take samples of the neighborhood noise. Notice the space between houses. Does the bedroom of that new house back up against someone else's porch, barbecue area, basketball court? Does the neighbor's dog bark every time someone walks by? Ask other tenants or homeowners whether the neighbors are considerate about keeping noise to a minimum.

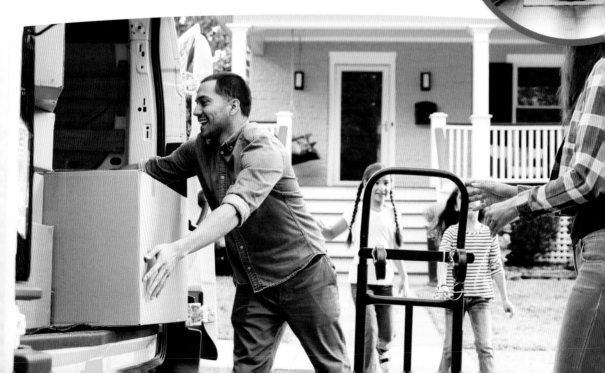

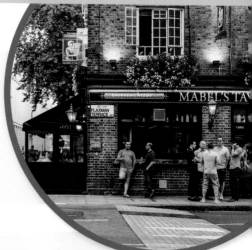

• Check noise levels around the area in the daytime, the evening, and at night. That quaint tavern or nearby park may seem quiet during the day, but what about late in the evenings or on weekends?

• When renting an apartment or buying a condo, check the thickness of the walls. Can you hear the television of the tenants next door?

• Check out the traffic patterns in the area. The bus stop near the front door may seem very convenient until you realize the whole apartment shakes each time the bus rumbles through on its 24-hour route. The same may be true if the home is located along a truck route. The house may be miles from the local airport, but takeoff and landing patterns may channel flights right over it.

• Be alert that high prices and fancy addresses are no guarantee of peace and quiet. Obviously, you cannot eliminate all the noise or find a place that meets all your noise-related criteria, but you should at least think about whether your new home will be a place where you can get some rest.

Chapter 5: Common Sleep Problems

SOME FOLKS DON'T GET ENOUGH SLEEP simply because they don't allow enough time in their daily lives to get a full night's sleep. Indeed, when schedules get tight and people get busy, sleep time is too often the first thing cut, as if sufficient shut-eye were a luxury rather than a necessity. But there are also plenty of adults who can't seem to get the sleep they need no matter how much time they block out for it. According to the National Sleep Foundation, nearly 75 percent of U.S. adults have some problem with sleep at least a few nights a week.

Sure, everyone occasionally misses out on a good night's sleep. But for a substantial portion of our population, an entire night of restful or uninterrupted sleep is something they only daydream about.

More than 70 classified sleep disorders affect between 50 and 70 million Americans.

The four most common sleep disorders are insomnia, sleep apnea, restless legs syndrome, and narcolepsy. Other sleep problems include chronic insufficient sleep, hypersomnias (excessive daytime sleepiness), circadian rhythm disorders (problems sticking to a regular sleep schedule), and parasomnias (abnormal sleep behaviors).

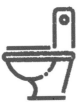

WHAT'S MY SLEEP PROBLEM?

Answer "yes" or "no" to the following questions. For anything you answer with a "yes," match the question number to the list on page 84 to identify the sleep disorder that might apply to you.

1. When you get in bed at night, do you often have trouble falling asleep? _____

2. Does it seem like you just can't fall asleep until very late at night? _____
3. Do you find it very difficult to wake up before 10 a.m.? _____
4. Do you tend to fall asleep early in the evening and wake up before the sun comes up? _____
5. Do you find yourself waking up several times throughout the night? _____

6. Do you wake up earlier in the morning than you need to and have trouble falling back to sleep? _____
7. Do you ever wake up in the night screaming, yelling, crying, or in an otherwise terrified state without knowing why? _____
8. Have you ever just collapsed on the spot the instant after hearing a funny joke, seeing a great sports play, or otherwise being excited? _____
9. Have you ever been told that you snore loudly and seem to stop breathing temporarily during the night? _____
10. Have you been told that you walk in your sleep? _____
11. Have you ever awoken to find yourself out of bed without remembering how you got there? _____
12. Have you been told that you move a lot in your sleep? _____
13. Have you ever injured yourself or anyone else while you were sleeping? _____

14. Do you feel tingly, prickly, itchy, or otherwise uncomfortable feelings in your legs as you start to fall asleep? _____

QUESTION/POSSIBLE SLEEP DISORDER

1. Insomnia or circadian rhythm disorder
2. Insomnia or circadian rhythm disorder
3. Circadian rhythm disorder
4. Circadian rhythm disorder
5. Insomnia
6. Insomnia or circadian rhythm disorder
7. Night terrors
8. Narcolepsy
9. Sleep apnea
10. Sleepwalking
11. Sleepwalking, night terrors, or REM sleep behavior disorder
12. Restless legs syndrome, periodic limb movement disorder, or REM sleep behavior disorder
13. Night terrors or REM sleep behavior disorder
14. Restless legs syndrome

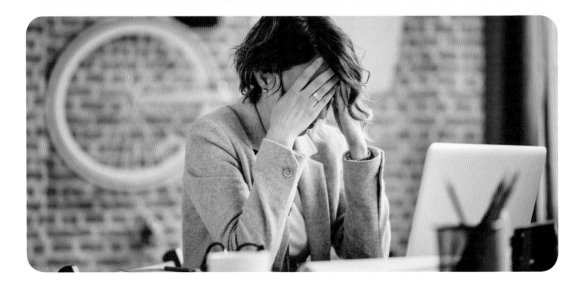

SLEEP APNEA

Ken chronically complains about being tired. He began having severe fatigue when he was in his early thirties. Up to that time, he had been a successful business owner. Since that time, however, he has lost his business and can't keep a job for more than a month. Of the numerous jobs he has held, nearly all have resulted in him getting fired for "laziness." Employers see his five to ten mini-naps each day as evidence he doesn't care about his job. His being very overweight and having other health conditions have led several doctors to misdiagnose the reason for his sleepiness. After several years and countless trips to different doctors who gave differing diagnoses, he recently went to a sleep disorders clinic, where they correctly diagnosed his condition as sleep apnea.

Ken is one of at least 25 million Americans who suffer from sleep apnea, a potentially life-threatening disorder that causes a person to stop breathing during sleep. Sleep apnea can strike people of any age, but is most frequently seen in men over 40, especially those who are overweight or obese. The word apnea means "without breath."

Because people who have sleep apnea frequently go from deeper sleep to lighter sleep during the night, they rarely spend enough time in deep, restorative stages of sleep. Not only do people with sleep apnea struggle with constant fatigue, but they are also at greater risk for accidents, high blood pressure, heart attacks, and other health conditions.

Children can also have sleep apnea, though they often present with different symptoms. See chapter 6 for more about children and sleep apnea.

TYPES OF SLEEP APNEAS

• **OBSTRUCTIVE SLEEP APNEA** occurs when the airway collapses or becomes blocked during sleep.

• **CENTRAL SLEEP APNEA** occurs when the brain fails to send proper signals to the muscles that control breathing.

• **COMPLEX OR MIXED SLEEP APNEA** is a combination of the two conditions. Breathing interruptions result from both airway obstruction and faulty brain signaling.

OBSTRUCTIVE SLEEP APNEA (OSA)

The most common form of sleep apnea is called obstructive sleep apnea (OSA). In obstructive sleep apnea, the throat muscles and tongue relax during sleep, and the tongue and uvula (the small dangling tissue at the back of the throat) sag and block the

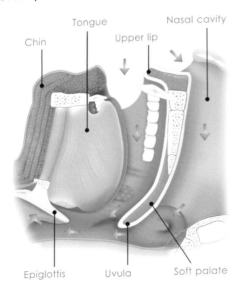

Open airway during sleep

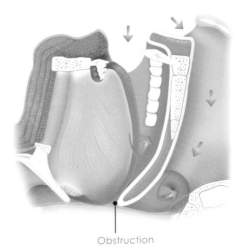

Sleep apnea present with obstruction

airway. Excess fatty tissue in the neck aggravates this by reducing the size of the airway, allowing it to collapse or be sucked closed. When the airway is either completely or partially blocked, breathing typically ceases for 10 to 20 seconds and, in some cases, for as much as a few minutes at a time. When breathing stops or becomes insufficient, it triggers a signal to the brain to jump-start the breathing again. But to do this, the brain has to awaken the body from deep sleep. The signal that the jump-start has kicked in is usually a loud snort and/or gasp. Most people do not even notice or remember this brief awakening. This impairment of breathing can occur up to 30 times an hour throughout the night, which significantly disrupts sleep cycles.

CENTRAL SLEEP APNEA (CSA)

In central sleep apnea (CSA), the pauses in breathing are caused by faulty brain signaling rather than a blocked airway. This condition is called central apnea because it's related to the function of the central nervous system. This less common type of sleep apnea occurs when the brain fails to transmit signals to breathing muscles. The breathing pauses typically last for 10 to 30 seconds and result in repeated awakenings during the night.

SLEEP APNEA SYMPTOMS

- Loud snoring
- Witnessed pauses in breathing during sleep
- Choking or gasping for breath during sleep
- Waking frequently to urinate
- Awakening groggy and unrested
- Excessive daytime sleepiness
- Morning headaches, dry mouth, or sore throat
- Lack of focus and concentration
- Learning or memory issues
- Irritability

DIAGNOSING SLEEP APNEA

Doctors diagnose sleep apnea based on medical and family histories, symptoms, a physical exam, and results from a sleep study (polysomnography) and/or other tests. Your doctor will determine if your sleep study should be conducted at a sleep center or at home with a portable diagnostic device. Polysomnography in a fully equipped sleep lab is regarded as the gold standard for diagnosing sleep apnea. A home study, especially if self-administered, is cheaper, but generally not sufficient to definitively diagnose sleep apnea.

OTHER TYPES OF SLEEP STUDIES

Other types of sleep studies include multiple sleep latency and daytime maintenance of wakefulness tests. Multiple sleep latency tests measure how quickly you fall asleep during a series of daytime naps and use sensors to record your brain activity and eye movements. A daytime maintenance of wakefulness test measures your ability to stay awake and alert.

SLEEP STUDIES (POLYSOMNOGRAPHY)

Sleep studies are noninvasive tests that help diagnose sleep apnea and other sleep disorders. A sleep study measures your sleep stages and cycles to identify if or when your sleep patterns are disrupted and why. Full sleep studies are usually done at a special sleep center, which is sometimes within a hospital.

If your doctor orders an overnight sleep study, you will arrive at the center in the evening and stay overnight. The test is performed in a bedroom similar to a hotel. After you get ready for bed, a specially-trained technologist will place removable sensors on your scalp, chin, chest, limbs, and the outer edge of your eyelids. Wires connect the sensors to a computer, but the wires are long enough to let you move normally in bed. A small clip also is placed on your finger or ear to monitor the level of oxygen in your blood. While you sleep, a technologist monitors your brain waves, eye movements, heart rate, breathing pattern, blood oxygen level, body position, limb movement, and snoring or any other noises you make. All of these measurements are recorded on a continuous graph.

In a split-night sleep study, a technologist will wake you up halfway through the night and fit you with a positive air pressure (PAP) device. This machine for sleep apnea has a tight-sealing nosepiece through which a gentle stream of air is delivered to enhance your breathing.

A sleep study generates a substantial amount of data, but the apnea-hypopnea index (AHI) is especially important for diagnosing obstructive sleep apnea. An apnea is when you stop breathing for 10 seconds or longer.

A hypopnea is when your breathing is partly blocked for 10 seconds or longer. The index number is the number of apneas and hypopneas experienced each hour.

The results of these tests will help your doctor determine if you have sleep apnea or another sleep disorder, and its severity. Your doctor will review your sleep study results with you and develop a treatment plan.

TREATING SLEEP APNEA

Common treatments for sleep apnea include lifestyle changes, breathing devices, mouthpieces, implants, and various surgical procedures. Lifestyle changes such as losing weight, quitting smoking, limiting alcohol, and sleeping on your side instead of your back may be all that's needed to treat mild sleep apnea. For moderate or severe sleep apnea, additional, more direct treatments are needed.

Continuous positive airway pressure (CPAP) is the most effective treatment for sleep apnea in adults. A CPAP machine uses mild air pressure to keep your airways open while you sleep. The machine delivers air to your airways through a specially designed nasal mask.

Most mouthpieces are custom-fit devices made by your dentist or orthodontist that you wear while sleeping. Mandibular repositioning mouthpieces cover the upper and lower teeth and hold the jaw in a position that prevents it from blocking the upper airway. Tongue retaining mouthpieces hold the tongue in a forward position to prevent it from blocking the upper airway. Some hybrid mouthpieces have features of both types. Mouthpieces are generally only used for mild sleep apnea.

SNORING VS. SLEEP APNEA

While loud and persistent snoring is a common symptom of sleep apnea, not everyone who snores has the sleep disorder. Almost half of all adults snore. While snoring without apnea may not be a health threat to the snorer, it may be a very real problem for a bed partner. Here are some stop-snoring tips:

- Sleep on your side.
- Lose weight.
- Avoid alcohol.
- Treat your allergies.
- Quit smoking.
- Buy an anti-snoring mouth guard.

HYPERSOMNIA

Hypersomnia disorders are characterized by recurrent episodes of excessive daytime sleepiness. People with a hypersomnia disorder may fall asleep at inappropriate times, such as at work, during a meal, or while driving. They may also have other sleep-related problems, a lack of energy, and difficulty thinking clearly. Narcolepsy is the most well known hypersomnia.

HYPERSOMNIA DISORDERS

- Narcolepsy
- Idiopathic hypersomnia
- Kleine-Levin syndrome
- Insufficient sleep syndrome

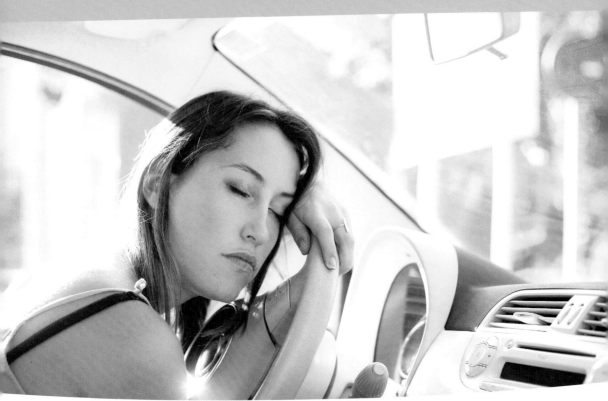

NARCOLEPSY

Narcolepsy is a hypersomnia disorder that affect's the brain's ability to control sleep-wake cycles. Individuals with narcolepsy suffer from excessive daytime sleepiness, even after adequate nighttime sleep. People with narcolepsy may unwillingly fall asleep during normal activities such as talking, eating, and even driving. These daytime "sleep attacks" can occur without warning and can last from a few seconds to more than 30 minutes. In between sleep attacks, individuals may have normal levels of alertness. People with narcolepsy may experience changes in normal REM sleep cycles, fragmented sleep, sudden muscle weakness while awake (cataplexy), vivid dreams and hallucinations, and sleep paralysis.

Cataplexy is an important symptom associated with narcolepsy. This sudden muscle

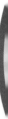

weakness is similar to the paralysis that normally occurs during REM sleep, but lasts a few seconds or minutes while the person is awake. Cataplexy tends to be triggered by sudden emotional reactions such as fear, laughter, anger, surprise, or joy. This may cause buckling of the knees, limpness at the neck, sagging facial muscles, or a complete body collapse.

Sleep paralysis is another symptom commonly associated with narcolepsy. People with narcolepsy may experience an inability to move or speak for a few moments. The paralysis occurs as the person is just falling asleep or waking up. Vivid or intense dreams can occur when people who have narcolepsy first fall asleep or wake up. The dreams are so lifelike that they can be confused with reality.

Narcolepsy usually begins in adolescence or early adulthood, and excessive sleepiness is almost always the first symptom. About one out of every ten people with narcolepsy has a close family member with the disorder, but most cases are not genetic. The exact cause of narcolepsy is still unknown, but research suggests that a substance in the brain called hypocretin plays a key role. Most people with narcolepsy have lower levels of hypocretin, which promotes wakefulness and regulates REM sleep.

After other medical conditions that can cause similar symptoms are ruled out, doctors may use an overnight sleep study (polysomnogram, or PSG) followed by a multiple sleep latency test (MSLT) to diagnose narcolepsy. Both tests reveal symptoms of narcolepsy—the tendency to fall asleep rapidly and enter REM sleep early, even during short naps.

Although there is no cure for narcolepsy, some of the symptoms can be treated with prescription medications, such as antidepressants and stimulants, and lifestyle changes. Stimulants are used to combat the severe daytime sleepiness, and antidepressants are used to control the cataplexy, sleep paralysis, and sleep-related hallucinations. Doctors usually also recommend taking brief naps throughout the day to help control excessive daytime sleepiness. Lifestyle changes discussed in chapters 2 and 3 can also help people with narcolepsy. These changes include avoiding smoking, caffeine, alcohol, and large meals before bed, exercising daily, maintaining a regular sleep schedule, and relaxing before bed.

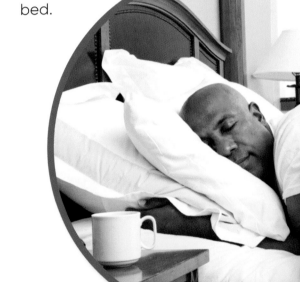

TYPES OF NARCOLEPSY

• **Type 1 narcolepsy** involves excessive daytime sleepiness, cataplexy, and a low hypocretin level.

• **Type 2 narcolepsy** is also characterized by excessive daytime sleepiness, but does not have cataplexy, sleep attacks, or a low level of hypocretin.

IDIOPATHIC HYPERSOMNIA

Idiopathic hypersomnia is a chronic neurological disorder marked by excessive daytime sleepiness and an insatiable need to sleep, despite adequate or prolonged nighttime sleep. Idiopathic (meaning "of unknown cause") hypersomnia is often mistaken for narcolepsy because the symptoms are similar. There is no FDA-approved treatment for idiopathic hypersomnia yet. But because narcolepsy and idiopathic hypersomnia share some of the same characteristics, certain medicines for narcolepsy may be prescribed "off-label" to help with the symptoms of idiopathic hypersomnia.

KLEINE-LEVIN SYNDROME

Kleine-Levin syndrome is a rare sleep disorder in the hypersomnia family that mainly affects adolescent males. Like other hypersomnias, Kleine-Levin syndrome involves excessive daytime sleepiness. Some people with Kleine-Levin syndrome experience increased appetite and hypersexuality along with the excessive sleeping. The disorder usually subsides on its own after several years.

INSUFFICIENT SLEEP SYNDROME

Insufficient sleep syndrome is a type of hypersomnia that occurs when a person regularly fails to get sufficient sleep at night. It results from decisions a person makes to forgo sleep in favor of other activities. Symptoms of insufficient sleep syndrome include regularly sleeping less than 6–8 hours per night, mood and behavior changes, excessive daytime sleepiness, lack of focus and concentration, memory problems, and lowered energy level.

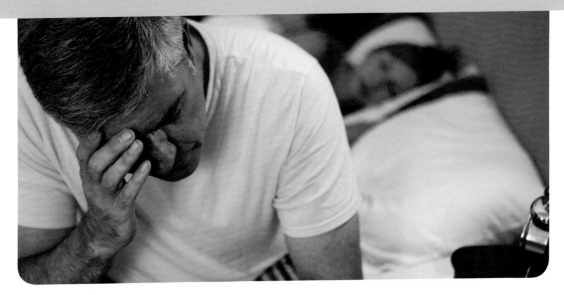

RESTLESS LEGS SYNDROME (RLS)

Restless legs syndrome (RLS), also called Willis–Ekbom disease, causes uncomfortable sensations in the legs and a powerful urge to move them. RLS sufferers describe feeling a crawling, burning, tingling, or prickling sensation in their legs when resting. These symptoms commonly occur in the evening and nighttime. They can also occur when sitting for long periods, such as while at a desk, watching a movie, or during long airplane or car trips. Moving the legs typically alleviates the discomfort, but the sensations often recur. Since symptoms usually worsen at night, RLS can make it difficult to fall asleep and stay asleep.

Many people with RLS also have periodic limb movements in sleep (PLMS), a condition characterized by involuntary jerking of the legs during sleep. PLMS can repeatedly awaken people who have RLS, reducing total sleep time and sleep quality.

Restless legs syndrome affects 5–15 percent of Americans. It can develop at any age, but is most common among middle-aged adults. Its prevalence increases with age. The disorder is more common in women than in men.

Doctors can usually diagnose restless legs syndrome based on self-reported symptoms and medical and family history. Some doctors may order a blood test to check iron levels or an overnight sleep study to monitor limb movements and rule out other sleep disorders.

In most cases, there is no known cause of restless legs syndrome. In other cases, RLS is caused by another condition, such as pregnancy, kidney failure, or iron deficiency anemia. Certain medications can aggravate RLS symptoms, including antinausea drugs, antipsychotic drugs, anti-depressants that increase serotonin, and cold and allergy medications that contain antihistamines.

Common treatments for RLS include behavioral changes, relaxation techniques, and prescription medication. Reducing use of caffeine, alcohol, and tobacco; regular exercise; and stretching, taking a hot bath, or massaging the legs before bedtime can improve symptoms. If iron or vitamin deficiency underlies RLS, symptoms may improve with iron, vitamin B_{12}, or folate supplements.

PERIODIC LIMB MOVEMENTS

Brief muscle twitches, jerking movements, or upward flexing of feet during sleep characterizes periodic limb movements in sleep (PLMS). These involuntary movements usually happen in the first half of the night during non-REM sleep. They cluster into episodes lasting anywhere from a few minutes to several hours. Within that time, movements tend to occur every 20–40 seconds. The movements themselves are not harmful, except perhaps to your bed partner. The main disadvantage is frequent waking, which can lead to daytime fatigue.

PARASOMNIAS

Parasomnias are sleep disorders that involve undesirable behaviors or events that occur while falling asleep, sleeping, or waking up. These include confusional arousals (partial awakenings from sleep during which people are confused), sleepwalking, night terrors, sleep paralysis, and REM sleep behavior disorder (acting out dreams). Most of these disorders—such as confusional arousals, sleepwalking, and night terrors—are more common in children, who tend to outgrow them. Chapter 6 contains more information on sleepwalking, night terrors, and nightmares in children.

PARASOMNIAS

- Night terrors
- Sleepwalking
- Confusional arousals
- Sleep paralysis
- Sleep talking (somniloquy)

- Bedwetting (enuresis)
- Sleep eating
- REM sleep behavior disorder (RBD)

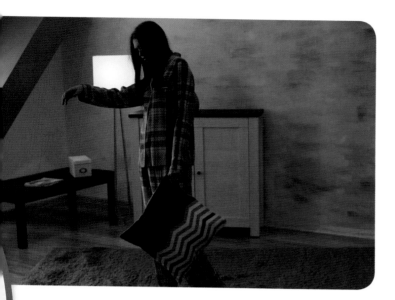

SLEEPWALKING

Sleepwalking, or somnambulism, is a type of parasomnia that occurs when a person gets up and walks around while asleep. During an episode, a sleepwalker may sit up with eyes wide open, get out of bed and walk around, perform routine tasks such as opening/closing doors or getting dressed, urinate in an inappropriate place, or injure themselves by bumping into objects or falling down stairs. They generally have no memory of their actions in the morning.

Sleepwalking usually occurs early in the night during deep non-REM sleep. Stress, fever, sleep deprivation, fatigue, and some medications are thought to trigger sleepwalking. Other causes include heredity, poor sleep hygiene, and sleeping with a full bladder.

Like many parasomnias, sleepwalking is more common in children than adults. In most cases, sleepwalking ends on its own after adolescence. Improving sleep hygiene, reducing tripping hazards in the sleep environment, and emptying the bladder before sleep can help manage sleepwalking for children and adults. Treatment for older children and adults may include stress-management techniques, hypnotherapy, or prescription medication.

It's a myth that you should never wake up a sleepwalker. When a family member sleepwalks, attempt to wake them up or gently guide them back to bed. Sleepwalkers may become combative if they are restrained.

NIGHT TERRORS

Night terrors (also called sleep terrors) are frightening instances in which a person screams, cries, even jumps from bed, while still fully asleep. These episodes can be very unsettling to the bed partner or others in the living situation and may result in bodily harm to the sleeper or others. The person may not awaken until the episode is over and may remember nothing of the incident.

You may recall that in non-REM sleep, physical movement is not restricted as it is in REM sleep. Since both sleepwalking and night terrors occur during non-REM sleep, the person can move about freely while still technically asleep. Night terrors are most common in the first third of the night.

Night terrors affect up to 40 percent of children and up to three percent of adults. Night terrors can be triggered by stress, fever, sleep deprivation, sleep schedule disruptions, sleeping in unfamiliar surroundings, or alcohol use. In children, this disorder usually disappears as they mature. Treatment for adult night terrors may include much of the same approaches that are used for adult sleepwalkers—hypnotherapy, psychotherapy, and stress-management techniques.

NIGHT TERRORS VS. NIGHTMARES

Night terrors occur in non-REM sleep, while nightmares (also called dream anxiety attacks) take place in REM. Dreaming typically only occurs in REM sleep, and when you are dreaming, your body is physically unable to move. So if you were having a nightmare, you wouldn't be able to grab that baseball bat stored in your bedroom closet to ward off your imagined attackers. The act of getting out of bed or verbally yelling or crying during sleep is more likely to be a night terror than a nightmare.

REM SLEEP BEHAVIOR DISORDER (RBD)

When a person has REM sleep behavior disorder (RBD), the body is not fully paralyzed during REM sleep. The dreamer is able to physically act out dramatic and/or violent dreams without waking. This, of course, can be very dangerous.

RBD is most common among middle-aged and older men, but the disorder also can occur in women and in younger people. Treatment involves medications and measures to protect the sleeper and others at night.

INSOMNIA

There are few things as frustrating as feeling tired and exhausted but being unable to sleep. You lie down in a nice, comfy bed at the end of the day, close your eyes, and . . . stay awake for hours. This maddening condition is insomnia.

Insomnia is a broad term that describes difficulty falling asleep, difficulty staying asleep, or waking up too early and not being able to return to sleep. In general, people with insomnia sleep less or sleep poorly despite having ample opportunity to sleep. Insomnia often causes problems during the day, such as extreme sleepiness, fatigue, difficulty concentrating, irritability, depressed mood, anxiety, forgetfulness, reduced motivation, and a lack of energy.

Half of all Americans experience occasional bouts of insomnia, and a good number experience it on a regular basis. Acute (short-term) insomnia affects all of us now and then. It can happen when we're worrying about an upcoming event, like a final exam or a big work

CAUSES OF CHRONIC INSOMNIA

• Depression, anxiety disorders, bipolar disorder, and post-traumatic stress disorder

• Neurological disorders, such as Parkinson's and Alzheimer's disease

• Thyroid dysfunction, arthritis, asthma, heartburn, or other medical conditions in which symptoms become more troublesome at night

• Other sleep disorders, such as sleep apnea, restless legs syndrome, periodic limb movements, and circadian rhythm disorders

• Various prescribed and over-the-counter medications that can disrupt sleep, such as decongestants, certain pain relievers, and steroids

• Sleep-disrupting behavior such consuming caffeine or alcohol late in the day, exercising shortly before bedtime, watching TV or reading while in bed, or irregular sleep schedules

• Menopause and hot flashes

• Enlarged prostate

presentation, grieving the loss of a loved one, or feeling distressed over bad news or events.

Chronic (long-term) insomnia occurs at least three nights per week for more than one month. Most cases of chronic insomnia are secondary, which means they are the symptom or side effect of some other problem, such as certain medical conditions, medications, and other sleep disorders. Sometimes chronic insomnia is the primary problem. Primary chronic insomnia is a distinct sleep disorder. Its cause is not yet well understood, but long-lasting stress, emotional upset, travel, and shift work may trigger primary chronic insomnia.

TYPES OF INSOMNIA

• Acute (short-term) insomnia can last from one night to a few weeks. Common causes include stress, family pressures, or a traumatic event.

• Chronic (long-term) insomnia occurs at least three nights per week for one month or longer. Most cases of chronic insomnia are secondary, due to another disorder or medicines. Primary chronic insomnia is not caused by something else.

DIAGNOSING INSOMNIA

Doctors diagnose insomnia based on sleep history (often by reviewing a sleep diary), medical history, and a physical exam. In some cases, your doctor may order a sleep study if another sleep disorder is suspected. Your doctor will also try to diagnose and treat any other underlying medical problems as well as identify behaviors that might be causing the insomnia.

TREATING INSOMNIA

Treatments for insomnia include lifestyle changes, counseling, and medicines. Lifestyle changes include avoiding substances such as caffeine, tobacco, stimulants, alcohol, and medicines that disrupt sleep, exercising early in the day, establishing bedtime routines, and making your sleep environment more sleep-friendly. A type of counseling called cognitive-behavior therapy (CBT) can help relieve the anxiety linked to chronic insomnia. For example, relaxation techniques and biofeedback are used to reduce anxiety. CBT works as well as prescription medicine for many people with chronic insomnia. For people with insomnia and major depression, CBT combined with antidepressants has shown promise in relieving both conditions.

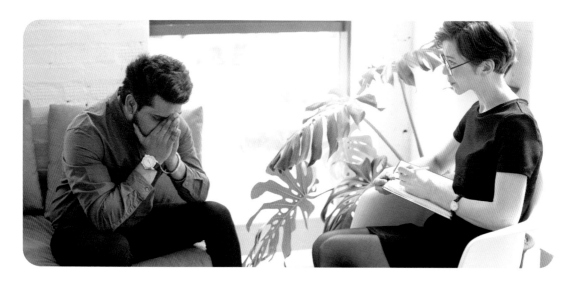

INSOMNIA CAUSED BY MEDICAL CONDITIONS

Many medical conditions can cause insomnia. Anyone who experiences pain, discomfort, stress, or limited mobility from medical problems knows all too well how their sleep can be affected. In addition to the physical pain or discomfort chronic conditions cause, prescribed medication for the condition may also contribute to poor sleep. Let's take a look at some of the most common medical conditions that can disrupt sleep and explore what you can do to minimize that effect. Prescription and over-the-counter medicines for insomnia are covered in chapter 7.

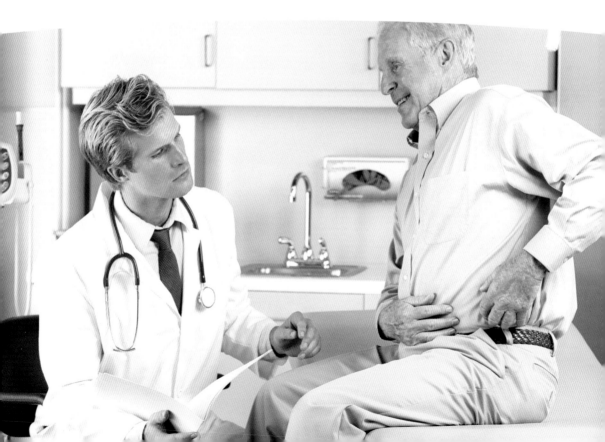

HEARTBURN

Heartburn happens when the esophagus, the tube that connects the mouth to the stomach, is exposed to the highly acidic contents of the stomach. When this occurs, the material in the stomach is said to "reflux," or back up, into the esophagus. This strong acid in the esophagus causes the burning sensation. In addition to the burning, or sometimes in its absence, you may have a bitter taste in your mouth and intense coughing fits, both due to the acid.

Reflux is most likely to occur when you are lying down. In this position, the force of gravity does not help move food from the stomach into the small intestine, where it is supposed to go. Because we generally sleep in a horizontal position, reflux is most common at night. Sleep apnea may also cause reflux through a siphoning effect that pulls stomach contents up into the esophagus.

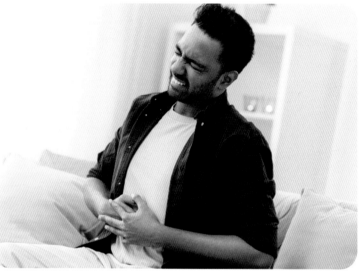

One technique that may help is to elevate your head at night to allow gravity to work for you. You can do this by placing bricks under the bedposts at the head of the bed, place several pillows under your head and shoulders to raise your upper body during sleep, or using an electrically adjustable bed, similar to the ones used in hospitals. If apnea is the cause of your heartburn, it needs to be treated.

EXCESSIVE NIGHTTIME URINATION

Nighttime trips to the bathroom may simply mean you consumed too much fluid in the evening. And, certainly, the need to urinate once during a night's sleep is not cause for concern. But needing to urinate two or more times every night requires investigation.

Numerous trips each night, combined with the time it takes to return to sleep, may add up to a significant amount of lost sleep over time. This pattern could also signal a medical problem. Excessive urination at night (called nocturia) is a common symptom of several conditions, including diabetes. In men, an enlarged prostate gland (a problem that occurs in most men as they age) is often the problem. An enlarged prostate can also be a warning sign of prostate cancer and should be evaluated promptly. In women, urinary tract infections frequently cause nocturia. Sleep apnea can also cause nocturia.

Drinking alcohol in the evening can be a factor in nocturia. And many prescription drugs have nocturia as a side effect. Because nocturia has so many causes, a doctor's evaluation is important. Afterward, your doctor may refer you to a urologist or other specialist.

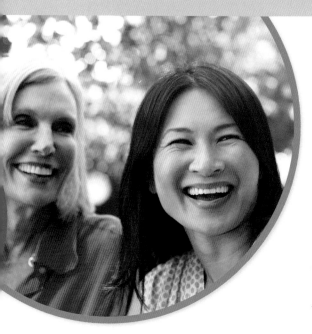

PREGNANCY

Pregnancy can temporarily interfere with restful sleep for a number of reasons. These include increased need to urinate during the night, nausea and/or heartburn, the baby's kicking, leg cramps and restless legs syndrome, and discomfort in many sleeping positions, especially in the third trimester.

Most, if not all, of these symptoms associated with pregnancy will stop once the baby is delivered. But it is after delivery, of course, when the real sleep deprivation begins, at least for a while. The best treatments for sleep-disruptive nightly feedings are frequent naps and lots of helping hands.

MENOPAUSE

As women approach menopause, hormone levels begin to shift. This shifting causes an imbalance between the female hormones estrogen and progesterone and is responsible for an increase in sleep disturbances. Hormonal fluctuations can cause insomnia indirectly as a result of frequent hot flashes and night sweats during menopause. Hormone replacement therapy has improved the sleeping patterns of many women. In addition, some women have found dietary changes and natural remedies to be helpful.

MENTAL HEALTH AND INSOMNIA

Sleep and mental health have a complex relationship. Mental health issues such as depression, anxiety, and bipolar disorder can cause insomnia. The reverse is also true: Insomnia and poor sleep can cause depression, anxiety, and other mental health issues. Sometimes both occur at once, resulting in a very difficult cycle to break. Understanding the possible connection between sleep disorders and mental health disorders can help you get to the root of both problems.

Depression and anxiety are two of the most common mental health disorders that interfere with sleep. Some of the typical symptoms of each condition are shown on page 110. If you believe that a mental health disorder is affecting your sleep and the symptoms persist for more than three weeks, seek professional help.

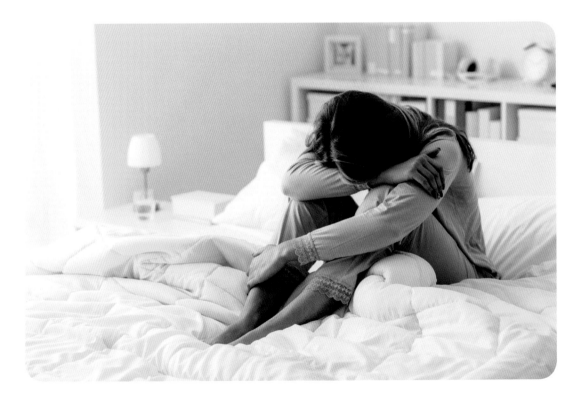

There are many types of depression and variations on the way it can affect sleep patterns. Here are a few.

MAJOR DEPRESSION: People with major depression feel sad, hopeless, and even suicidal through much of the day. People with major depression often have trouble falling asleep, staying asleep, and have excessive daytime sleepiness.

DYSTHYMIA: This is a milder form of major depression, also associated with fragmented sleep and excessive sleep. People with dysthymia experience fewer symptoms than people with major depression and in a less intense way, but symptoms typically persist much longer.

BIPOLAR DISORDER: People with bipolar disorder swing between extreme highs (manic episodes) and lows (depressive episodes). When they're manic, they're overly energetic and unable to sleep. When they're depressed, they oversleep and have daytime fatigue.

SEASONAL AFFECTIVE DISORDER (SAD): SAD is a type of seasonal depression. It is more prevalent during the winter months, when there are fewer hours of available sunlight. Symptoms include fatigue, excessive sleep, worsened mood, and cravings for carbs and candy. Therapy using a special light box has proven helpful for many people with SAD.

SYMPTOMS OF DEPRESSION

- Feeling of sadness, hopelessness, despair
- Withdrawal from usual activities
- Sleeping more than usual
- Excessive daytime sleepiness
- Difficulty concentrating
- Insomnia
- Lack of energy
- Low self-esteem
- Weight gain or loss

SYMPTOMS OF ANXIETY

- Racing heart
- Sweating palms
- Muscle tension
- Shortness of breath
- Irritability
- Frequent decision-making paralysis
- Trouble maintaining focus and concentration
- Worrying about worst-case scenarios
- Racing or obsessive thoughts
- Difficulty falling sleep
- Frequent waking in the night

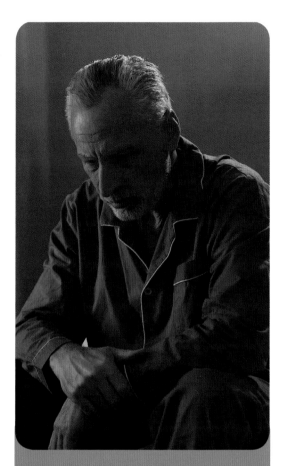

THE DEPRESSION-INSOMNIA LINK

People with insomnia are ten times more likely to develop depression than people without. More than 75% of depressed individuals display insomnia symptoms. The good news is that treating either depression or insomnia tends to improve symptoms of the other.

CIRCADIAN RHYTHM DISORDERS

Remember circadian rhythms from chapter 1? The body has a sort of internal circadian pacemaker, or clock, centered in the brain. This clock governs things like appetite and sleep, taking cues from things like sunlight and darkness. But what if your lifestyle is out of sync with your body clock? Circadian rhythm disorders such as jet lag and shift work can be traced to the clash between body clock and lifestyle.

The body clock can be stubborn and difficult to change. Just because you all of a sudden change the hours at which you eat doesn't mean your body will automatically feel hungry at the new times. Likewise, just because you switch from a day job to a job that keeps you working until 2 a.m. doesn't mean your body will automatically adjust to your new bedtime or wake-up time.

People with circadian rhythm disorders have difficulty falling asleep or waking up at the right time, have trouble staying asleep, and may wake feeling unrefreshed. Symptoms of a circadian rhythm disorder include the inability to fall asleep or stay asleep, daytime fatigue, and poor concentration.

Treating circadian rhythm disorders often involves a combination of chronotherapy (gradually moving the bedtime up or back) and light therapy (exposing yourself to sunlight to reset the body clock and reinforce awake time). For example, if your body wants you to sleep late in the morning but your boss doesn't, try gradually moving your bedtime up and exposing yourself to bright sunlight in the early morning to help reset your sleep-wake cycle.

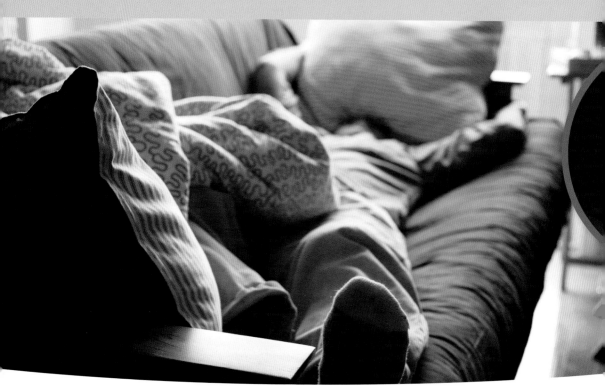

JET LAG

Those who travel across multiple time zones have likely felt the effects of jet lag. Jet lag can cause disturbed sleep, daytime fatigue, indigestion, and a general feeling of discomfort. The severity of jet lag depends on the number of time zones crossed and the direction of travel. The farther you travel, the more severe the jet lag. Eastward travel generally causes more severe jet lag than westward travel because traveling east requires you to shorten the day, and your biological clock is better able to adjust to a longer day than a shorter day.

Jet lag can also be made worse by the airplane itself. Airplanes tend to have poorer air quality, lower humidity, and cramped conditions. Lower humidity results in dehydration, while being forced to sit still for a long flight makes the body achy.

Fortunately, jet lag is a temporary condition that does not usually require treatment. Some tips on dealing with jet lag follow.

- **PLAN AHEAD.** In the days or weeks leading up to your trip, gradually adjust your biological clock. For westward travel, move your bedtime and wake time 30 minutes later each day prior to your trip. For eastward travel, move your wake time 15 minutes earlier each day and try to advance your bedtime.

- **USE SUNLIGHT.** Sunlight is a powerful tool in resetting your biological clock. Decreasing light exposure at bedtime and increasing light exposure at wake time can help you make adjustments prior to your trip. When you arrive at your destination, spend a lot of time outdoors so your body gets the light cues it needs to adjust to the new time zone. If your destination doesn't have much natural sunlight, consider using light therapy.

- **AVOID ALCOHOL AND CAFFEINE.** These substances mess with your ability to fall asleep and stay asleep. Instead, drink plenty of water while you're flying.

- **USE MELATONIN.** Your body produces a hormone called melatonin that causes drowsiness and signals to the brain that it's time to fall asleep. Melatonin supplements are available over the counter. Try taking melatonin at local bedtime nightly until you have adapted to the time zone.

- **WHEN IN ROME.** Follow the same social schedule as other people at the destination. Engaging in the same activities at the same times as locals will help you adjust to local time.

SHIFT WORK

Bill works the night shift most of the time at the local plastics manufacturing plant. He starts work at 11:00 p.m. and gets off at 7:00 a.m., five days a week. On workdays he tries to sleep until about 3:00 p.m., but there always seem to be things that disrupt his sleep, so he feels tired a lot. On weekends, because he wants to spend time with his family, he attempts to sleep on their schedule, which doesn't work very well for him. Bill's body clock can't make any permanent adjustments because he is always switching his sleep between days and nights.

Shift work does not come naturally to us. Our bodies are designed to work in the daylight and on a consistent schedule. Working on artificial schedules with nighttime hours has consequences. People with shift work disorder can experience insomnia, excessive sleepiness and fatigue, headaches, irritability, and lack of concentration. These people tend to sleep poorly and have decreased alertness during waking hours. They also have more accidents (both work- and non-work-related), work less efficiently, and have increased stress at home.

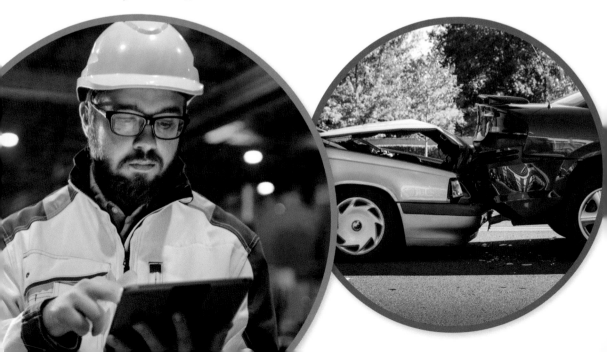

If you must work the night shift, here are some tips that might help:

• Determine a feasible sleep schedule that will enable you to get 7–9 hours of sleep on a daily basis. Be sure to share this schedule with your partner, family members, and/or roommates; minimizing disturbances and interruptions is key to an effective sleep schedule.

• Once you determine a sleep schedule, keep that as consistent as possible—even on weekends or other days off.

• No matter what time of day you sleep, make sure your sleep environment is dark, quiet, and temperature-controlled. Block outside noise by using earplugs or a white noise machine. Block sunlight with blackout curtains or shades, or cover your eyes with eyeshades.

• Expose yourself to bright lights whenever your 'day' begins and at your workplace. Consider using the type of bright-light box used to treat seasonal affective disorder (SAD) during your waking hours.

• By the same token, avoid bright lights when you are winding down and preparing to sleep. These measures help your circadian rhythm adjust to a shift work schedule, since the 24-hour cycle is largely influenced by daylight and darkness.

• If you work night shifts, consider taking vitamin D supplements. Vitamin D is a nutrient found in natural sunlight, and supplements can increase your wakefulness and boost overall immune health.

• Plan errands ahead, so they don't interfere with sleep. For example, if you sleep right after work, use a bank that has evening hours.

• Minimize your number of shift changes so that your body's biological clock has a longer time to adjust to a nighttime work schedule.

• Avoid taking overtime shifts or agreeing to work extended hours; the extra pay may be tempting, but long shifts only further increase your risk of a workplace accident.

• If you have a long commute, try carpooling with your coworkers; this will cut down on the amount you have to drive to and from work.

If you are unable to fall asleep during the day, and all else fails, talk with your doctor to see whether you're a candidate for short-acting prescription sleeping pills to help you sleep during the day.

ROTATING-SHIFT WORKERS

Rotating-shift workers face the biggest problems. Practice these strategies to make rotating-shift work easier:

1. Make it easier on your body by changing from one shift to another as infrequently as possible.
2. When you must change shifts, the change should occur in this order: day shift to swing shift to night shift. This order follows your body clock's natural tendency to move forward. If you shift in the other direction (day shift to night shift to swing shift), you will find it much harder to adapt to each shift rotation.

GETTING HELP

If you recognize your own sleep patterns or symptoms in any of the descriptions in this chapter, be sure to read through and try some of the suggestions in chapters 2–4 for improving sleep. If your sleep still does not improve, if you suspect you have a sleep disorder, or if you think another medical condition may be causing your sleep troubles, you should consult your doctor. In turn, your doctor may provide a referral to a sleep specialist or sleep clinic.

Prior to your first appointment with a sleep specialist, you will probably be asked to fill out a sleep questionnaire and complete a sleep log. At the first visit, the sleep specialist will review these and ask you a number of questions to try to understand the physical, psychological, and social issues that might be part of your sleep problem. To diagnose certain sleep disorders such as narcolepsy the sleep specialist may perform tests such as a multiple sleep latency test (MSLT) or

arrange an overnight sleep study (polysomnography) in the sleep lab so your sleep patterns can be monitored. Once a diagnosis has been made, the sleep specialist may discuss the findings and possible treatments with you or may relay that information to your regular doctor so that together you and your doctor can consider appropriate treatment options. You'll learn more about various self-help, pharmaceutical, and alternative treatments for sleep problems in the chapters to come.

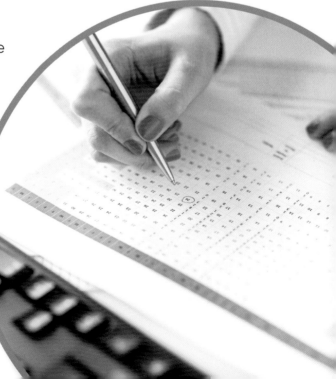

Chapter 6: Children and Sleep

AS ANY PARENT CAN TELL you, the quality and quantity of a baby's sleep affects the well-being of everyone in the home. The arrival of a baby generally means the departure of uninterrupted nights and lazy mornings sleeping in. And even after those first few months of nighttime feedings, you are still likely to be called upon in the middle of the night to chase a monster from under a bed, give a drink of water, or take a temperature every now and then.

Sacrificing sleep for a child's sake is part of being a caring and concerned parent. And some disruptions just come with the territory. But there are some tips and techniques you can try to help both you and your child get needed sleep. This chapter will help you determine how much sleep your child needs, how to respond when you're awakened in the middle of the night, and how to get your kids to sleep through the cries, screams, and avoidance tactics. We'll also cover some specific sleep problems that affect children.

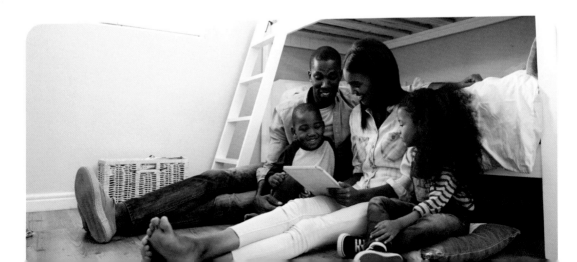

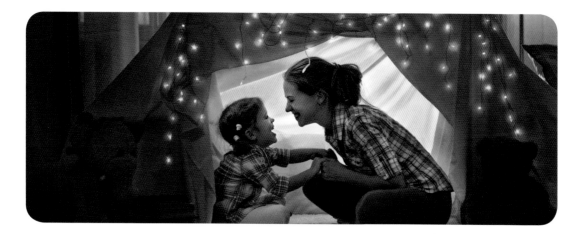

UNDERSTAND YOUR CHILD'S SLEEP NEEDS

Especially if you are a first-time parent, you may have all kinds of concerns about your child's sleep habits and needs. Should your newborn be sleeping so much? When, oh, when, will your baby start sleeping through the night? If your toddler resists your attempts to put him down for the night, does it mean you're putting him to bed too early?

Understanding the typical sleep needs and quirks at various ages may help allay some of your worries and help you encourage your child to get the sleep she needs. The chart on page 120 shows the average sleep needs of children at various ages to give you some insight. However, it's important to keep in mind that each child is unique. Some children may need more or less than these averages, and the amount of sleep they require at any particular time may be affected by a variety of factors in addition to age, such as growth spurts, changes in routine, illness, and stress.

To broaden your understanding, let's take a look at various stages in childhood and how patterns of sleep and wakefulness change.

HOW MUCH SLEEP DO CHILDREN NEED?

Age	Total average sleep time/day	Nap time
Birth to eight weeks	16–18 hours	Whenever not eating
Four months	15 hours	Frequent
Nine months	14 hours	Twice a day (1–2 hours)
One year	12-14 hours	Twice a day (1–2 hours)
18 months	12-13 hours	Once a day (afternoon)
Two to three years	12 hours	Once a day (afternoon)
Three to six years	10-12 hours	Once a day until age six years or so

BIRTH TO SIX MONTHS

In the beginning, most babies sleep most of the time—and that's what they're supposed to do. Along with eating, sleeping is essential for healthy development. Newborns sleep up to 18 hours a day, divided about equally between day and night. Newborns should be wakened every three to four hours for feedings until they have good weight gain. After that, it's okay if your baby sleeps for longer periods. By three months of age, babies typically sleep about 15 hours a day, with eight to nine hours at night (usually with an interruption or two) and two or three daytime naps. By six months, the average is about 14 hours a day, with two to three daytime naps. However, it is important to remember that there is great variability in sleep patterns among individual babies.

There is no set age at which all babies routinely begin sleeping through the night. At first, sleeping is tied closely to feeding—babies will tend to fall asleep when they're full and wake up when they're hungry. It isn't until about three to four months of age that being tired generally takes priority over being hungry. It is also at about three or four months that babies can stay awake for relatively longer stretches. Although your baby may start sleeping through the night—or at least for longer stretches at a time—somewhat earlier or later, you can reasonably expect to see this beginning to happen somewhere between three and four months of age.

SIX MONTHS TO ONE YEAR

During the second half of the first year, the sleep needs and patterns of babies become even more variable. Typically, babies will sleep approximately 10 to 12 hours during the night and take two naps during the day. The naps may last as little as 20 minutes or as long as

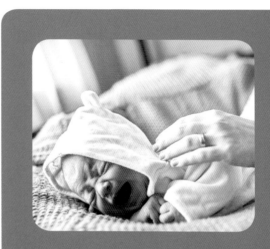

COLIC

Colic is frequent, prolonged, and intense crying in an infant. It's particularly frustrating for parents because it happens for no apparent reason and no amount of consoling seems to help. It often occurs during the evening when parents are often exhausted. The crying is unrelenting and forceful, and the infant may draw up or stiffen her legs, clench her fists, flail her arms, or arch her back. The exact cause of colic is unknown. It usually begins about three to six weeks after birth and is gone by four months. Up to 40 percent of all infants have colic.

a couple of hours. If your baby's sleep needs were on the high end in the first six months, the same will likely be true during the second half of the first year, and vice versa.

You can try to influence your baby's schedule by determining the length of naps and the timing of meals, but usually your baby will sleep when he's sleepy and eat when he's hungry. Depending on your child-raising philosophy, you can remain flexible or try to alter your baby's schedule to better fit in with the family's schedule. If he's going to sleep two to three hours later than you'd like, you'll probably want to try shortening one of his daily naps. If your baby is sleeping too long at one nap time, you might shorten the next one. He may fall asleep more easily at the preferred bedtime, or he may be overly tired and cry and fuss at you longer. You might

also try to stimulate and play with him more during awake periods; this may help him use up enough energy so that he's tired enough to fall asleep when you want him to. You don't, however, want to overstimulate your baby just before bedtime. Your baby needs a little quiet time before he can fall asleep.

What to do if your baby wakes you up at night because he's wet and then doesn't want to go back to sleep? Try changing his diaper just before bed; that may help him get through the night. You might also try adding a blanket or using a sleeper to keep him warmer; it could be the cold more than the dampness that wakes him. When you do change him, be as brief as possible. Let him know it's time for sleeping. If he cries once his diaper has been changed, it's okay. If you allow him to keep you awake just to play, you reinforce his awake time, and he'll expect the same treatment in the future.

If your baby wakes in the middle of the night, sometimes he just needs a few minutes to settle down on his down. If he's not sick, and he doesn't settle down on his own, comfort him without picking him up. You can talk or sing softly to your baby, rub his back, then leave him to settle down again on his own. The goal is for babies to fall asleep on their own and learn to soothe themselves back to sleep if they wake up in the middle of the night.

TODDLERS (1–3 YEARS)

Most toddlers sleep 12 to 14 hours over a 24-hour period. At one year of age, most toddlers will still require two naps a day, but by two-and-a-half, many get by with only one. The transition is not always smooth, and your toddler may experience an awkward period at around 18 months of age—two naps may be too much, yet one won't quite be enough.

You can get clues about the number and length of naps that are appropriate from your child herself. When your toddler is tired, she might take her blanket and head for bed, tell you she wants a nap, or simply stop what she's doing and fall asleep. In such cases, you should let her nap. If, on the other hand, she's happily and busily playing, you can probably let her skip a nap. But it's important to schedule some quiet time, even if your toddler chooses not to sleep.

You may find that, even after weeks or months of sleeping through the night, your child starts waking up and crying in the middle of the night

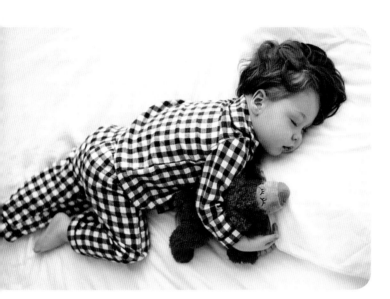

for no apparent reason. Your child may be experiencing separation anxiety—she may need to check to be sure you are really still there. These unhappy awakenings will eventually stop. Keep the time you spend with her when she does wake up short. Comfort her and make sure that there's not something bothering her physically (such as a wet or dirty diaper, a cold room, or an empty stomach). Try putting a night-light in her room and making sure a favorite toy or blanket is within reach. If she awakens again, go to her but don't pick her up;

leave her in her crib as you pat her and tell her that everyone else is sleeping. If she continues to wake you up, comfort her from the doorway of her room; let her see you, and tell her that everything is fine but that it's time for sleeping. Finally, if it continues, just call to her from your room and reassure her that everything's all right. Eventually, she will learn that while you love her and care about her, it's time for sleeping.

PRESCHOOLERS (3–5 YEARS)

The sleep needs of preschoolers vary enormously. Typically, however, preschoolers sleep about 11 to 12 hours per night. Although some younger preschoolers require a short afternoon nap, by age five, most no longer need a nap. Instead, they may benefit from some quiet time midday or in the afternoon. Many preschools have quiet periods when children lie on mats or just rest. As preschoolers give up naps, they may go to bed at night earlier than they did as toddlers.

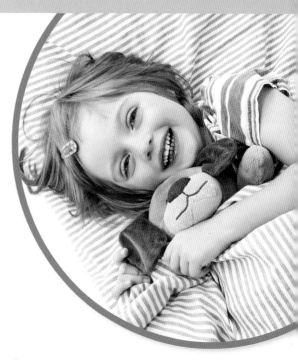

SCHOOL-AGED KIDS (6–12 YEARS)

School-age kids need 10 to 11 hours of sleep per night. But homework, sports, afterschool activities, family schedules, and increased exposure to electronic media can contribute to kids not getting needed sleep. Lack of sleep may have a direct effect on children's health, development, and behavior. Consistent bedtimes are important. Leave enough time before lights-out to allow your child to unwind. Switch off the electronics at least an hour before bed and keep TVs, gaming systems, computers, and other devices out of their bedrooms.

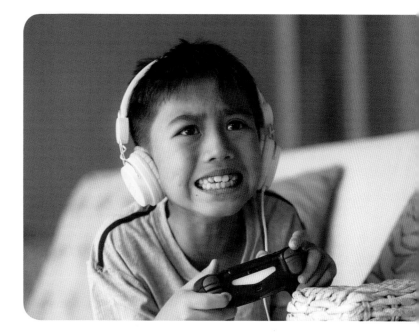

TEENS (13–18 YEARS)

Teens need about nine to ten hours of sleep per night, but most don't get it. The hormonal changes that occur during puberty tend to shift adolescents' biological clock so that teenagers are more likely to want to go to bed later and wake up later than younger children and adults. This delayed sleep-wake rhythm conflicts with the early-morning start times of many schools. Homework, friends, after-school activities, part-time jobs, electronics, and early start times lead to many teenagers being chronically sleep deprived. Tired teens find it difficult to concentrate, learn, or even stay awake in class. Sleep deprivation can also result in short-term memory loss, delayed response time, behavioral problems, and mood swings.

Ideally, your teenager should go to bed at the same time each night and get up at the same time each morning, allowing for at least nine hours of sleep. Nixing afterschool naps, curbing caffeine use, turning off the TV and other electronics an hour before bedtime, and practicing relaxation techniques can help teenagers improve sleep.

ESTABLISH A BEDTIME ROUTINE

No matter what your child's age, establishing a bedtime routine will encourage good sleep habits. Think back to the purpose of bedtime routines we suggested for adults. A bedtime routine gradually tells your mind and body that it's time for sleep. That's exactly what you seek to accomplish for your child in establishing a bedtime routine. The routine you set up also puts sleep patterns into place that your child may follow for many years.

When setting up the bedtime routine, keep two things in mind:

1. Leave plenty of time to walk through the routine without hurrying. End your time together calmly and quietly. Rushing through the routine or pushing your child to hurry defeats the purpose of the routine. In addition, never send your child to bed as a punishment; it only fosters negative associations with bed and bedtime.

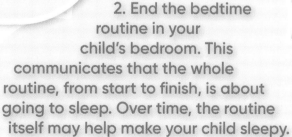

2. End the bedtime routine in your child's bedroom. This communicates that the whole routine, from start to finish, is about going to sleep. Over time, the routine itself may help make your child sleepy.

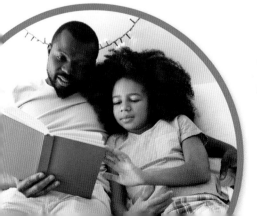

It may not be necessary to go through the entire sleep routine at naptime. You should abbreviate the routine to one or two items such as reading one story or listening to one song. While some children can nap anywhere, others may feel more secure in their own bed. It might help to give her something familiar to sleep with such as the stuffed animal or blanket she uses at night. Whenever possible, encourage your child to nap at about the same time each day. This helps establish and reinforce a regular wake-sleep rhythm.

WHAT TO INCLUDE IN BEDTIME ROUTINES

Every child will have a slightly different bedtime ritual. It doesn't have to take a long time, but it should include a winding-down period. The routine should be done consistently and in the same order each night. Here are two sample routines:

- Have a bath (or wash up), put pajamas on, brush teeth, read a story, go to the bathroom, choose a stuffed animal for sleeping, get tucked in with a kiss.

- Have a light snack, play a quiet game, wash face, brush teeth, put pajamas on, listen to a song, get tucked in with a kiss.

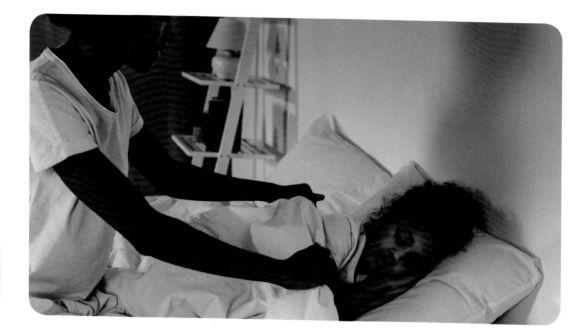

BE STRICT ABOUT BEDTIME

No parent has been spared their child's bedtime plea to stay up "just five more minutes." When the attempts to stay up past bedtime are infrequent or for special occasions, they don't indicate a real problem. Allowing your child a rare night up past his regular bedtime is generally harmless. However, when a child repeatedly puts up a fight at bedtime, you need to put your foot down. You are responsible for his health and well-being, and getting plenty of sleep is essential for a growing child.

First, determine a good bedtime for your child. Not every child needs exactly the same amount of sleep. So observe over time the amount of sleep that allows your child to function well. Then, make getting him to bed on time a priority. Resist the distractions that can delay you in this mission: Open the mail later, don't answer that text, and leave the dishes. Schedule evening activities so that you have adequate time to make bedtime pleasant, relaxing, and nurturing for your child. His need for gentle coaxing through his bedtime routine is an excellent reason for you to slow down, really listen, and engage with him emotionally.

If a relative, babysitter, or other caretaker watches your child, keep your child's bedtime routine the same. Be sure to inform the caretaker of the pre-sleep routine and the approximate time it should begin and end. When children shuttle between parents, make deliberate efforts to agree upon a bedtime routine and bedtime that are consistent at both homes.

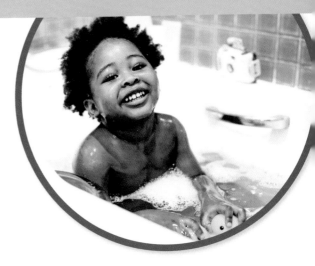

HELP TODDLERS TRANSITION

Saying goodbye is hard for children. When they can't see you, they think you are gone and may never

come back, even though you may be in the next room. This is called separation anxiety, and it can often strike at bedtime or during the night.

To help ease your child's anxiety, try giving her a transitional object. This transitional object, usually a blanket or stuffed animal,

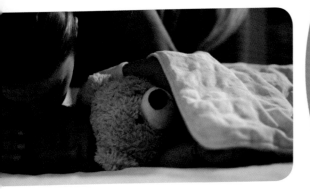

can help her feel more secure as she makes the transition from being with you to being without you. Some studies have shown that even an item of clothing that a child has frequently seen her mother wearing and that has her mother's scent can be an effective transitional object to aid sleep. Indeed, your child may become so attached to the transitional object that she takes it wherever she goes. To your child, the object is uniquely important because it provides comfort and security. When you wash it, don't be surprised if she sits at the dryer waiting for the final cycle to finish.

Although the value of the transitional object goes beyond aiding sleep, that is one of its most important functions. Your child must learn to fall asleep without your physical presence. Also, when your child awakens in the night, she must learn to return to sleep without calling for you each time. The transitional object can help a great deal.

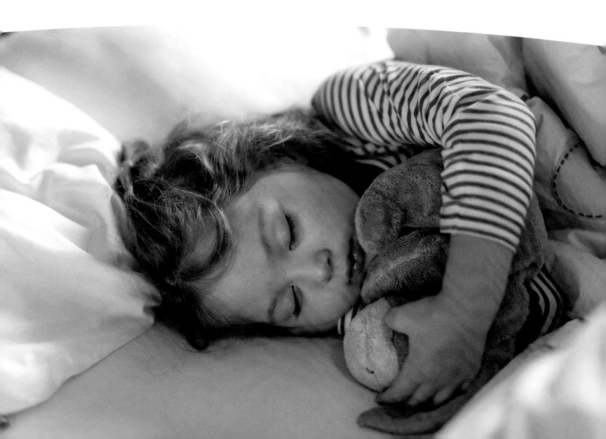

SPECIFIC SLEEP PROBLEMS

Some sleep problems in children can be easily resolved, while others can take more time and effort. Here are a few of the most common sleep problems among children.

SLEEPWALKING

Sleepwalking in children is extremely common because their sleep is so deep. When something happens to arouse them in the night, the part of their brain responsible for waking them cannot easily overcome the part responsible for sleep. The result is a state in which the child is partly awake and partly asleep.

Children sleepwalk with their eyes open and can see objects around them. But, they may misinterpret what they see. A window might look like a door, and the child might attempt to climb out. While children are usually able to go up and down stairs while sleepwalking, they may do so clumsily, and a fall could result. Therefore, if your child sleepwalks, it's important to protect her by locking windows, blocking stairways (with a safety gate, for example), and removing hazardous objects from her immediate vicinity.

Children who walk in their sleep generally do not need medical attention. Most children outgrow the problem by early adolescence. Parents need only know how to handle sleepwalking episodes when they do occur. Contrary to popular belief, waking a sleepwalking child is not dangerous. But, a child who awakens suddenly in strange surroundings may become frightened and confused. It is usually not necessary to wake a sleepwalking child. Most times, you can gently guide your child back to bed. Be persistent but not forceful or confrontational. The child will probably have no memory of the episode in the morning.

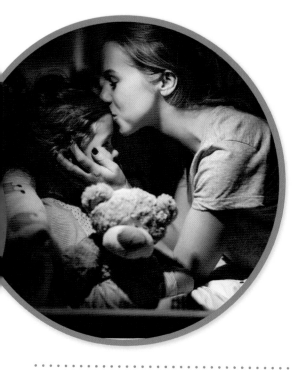

NIGHT TERRORS

As with sleepwalking, night terrors occur when a child is in deep sleep. The child screams loudly, disturbing any nearby sleepers. At times, the child may even dash out of bed screaming. The techniques for handling night terrors are the same as for coping with sleepwalking: Protect the child from danger, carry on as few exchanges as possible, and guide the child back to bed. Don't ask the child to tell you why he is screaming or carrying on: He doesn't know, often cannot answer at all, and will just get more agitated if you try to arouse him from this state.

Parents may worry that something is wrong with a child who experiences night terrors. Unless the terrors occur frequently, this is generally not the case. Night terrors are more common in children younger than five, and in most cases, eventually cease without treatment. If your child experiences a night terror, simply go to him, rub his back, offer gentle words of assurance, and guide him back to bed. He will not remember the episode in the morning. You can return to sleep knowing night terrors are fairly common and usually do not require medical attention.

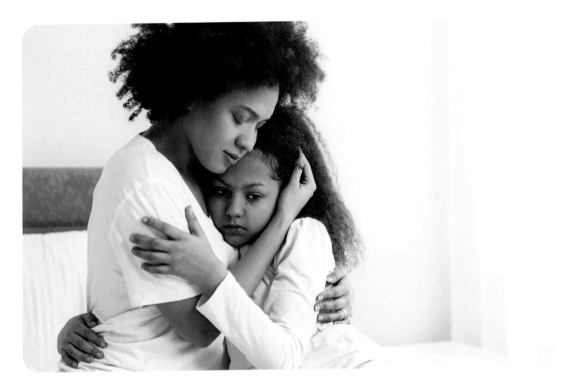

NIGHTMARES

Nightmares are scary dreams that can wake your child and leave her upset and needing comfort. After a nightmare, she may be afraid of going back to sleep or being left alone. She is not yet able to tell the difference between a dream and reality and may fear that what she saw in her dream will actually happen. Knowing this, the best thing you can do for a child awakened by a nightmare is to comfort her—hold her, stroke her hair, reassure her, perhaps even turn on a light to reinforce the difference between her nightmare and reality. Try to be patient: It may take a while for her to fall back to sleep, and she may need the reassurance of your presence until she does.

Nightmares are often confused with night terrors, but they are not the same. Night terrors usually occur during the first couple of hours of sleep. The child never fully awakens during a night terror, so she is likely to fall back asleep easily once it's over and won't remember it the next day. In contrast, nightmares typically occur after a child has been asleep for several hours. The nightmare wakes the child, so she is likely to need comforting and may have trouble falling back to sleep.

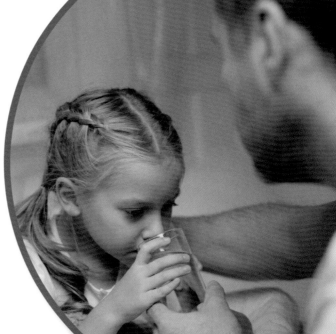

AVOIDING NIGHTMARES

There's no foolproof method for stopping all nightmares, but there are some sound steps you can take to try to keep them from happening with any frequency.

- Don't read, watch, or tell scary stories.
- Be responsive to your child's fears. Reassure her of your protection and presence when she wakes up after a nightmare.
- Help ensure that she regularly gets enough sleep, since lack of sleep can cause more dreaming and nightmares.
- Try to determine if your child is experiencing an unusual amount of stress during the day, and do what you can to alleviate it. If your child starts having nightmares with some regularity, stress may be the cause. If you can't remove the source of the stress, do your best to support and reassure your child.

SLEEP APNEA

Sleep apnea is typically thought of as a sleep disorder that affects adults, but it also affects children. Sleep apnea in adults and children is a serious condition in which airflow is partially or totally obstructed many times throughout sleep.

COMMON SYMPTOMS OF APNEA DURING SLEEP INCLUDE:

- Pauses in breathing.
- Snoring. Most, but not all, children with sleep apnea snore.
- Noisy or difficult breathing.
- Breathing through the mouth.
- Coughing or choking.
- Disturbed sleep. Breathing pauses often briefly awaken the child, causing restless sleep and daytime sleepiness.

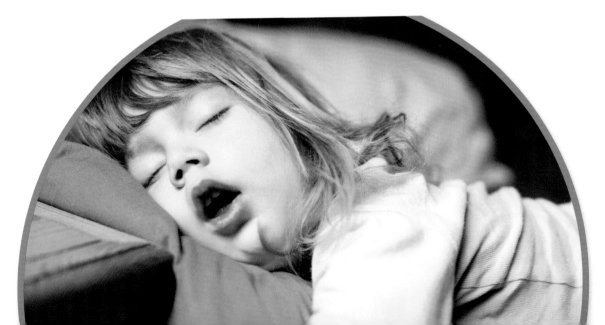

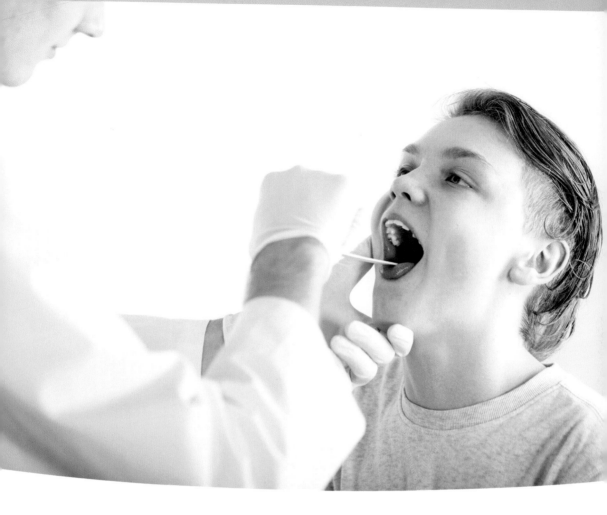

The cause of sleep apnea in most children is enlarged adenoids and tonsils. Once the muscles in the child's neck relax during sleep, the tonsils and adenoids block the airway. Treatment typically involves removal of the tonsils and adenoids. If allergies are the cause, these need to be identified and controlled. Weight loss may eliminate sleep apnea in overweight children. There is also a special mask that can be worn by the child to keep the air passage open during sleep.

RISK FACTORS FOR SLEEP APNEA IN CHILDREN

The following traits or conditions put a child at higher risk for sleep apnea:

- Enlarged tonsils or adenoids.
- Frequent ear infections, sore throats, tonsillitis, and allergies.
- Being overweight.
- A small, receding chin. This may indicate a smaller airway.
- Down syndrome. Children with Down syndrome may have several problems with their airway that obstruct breathing.

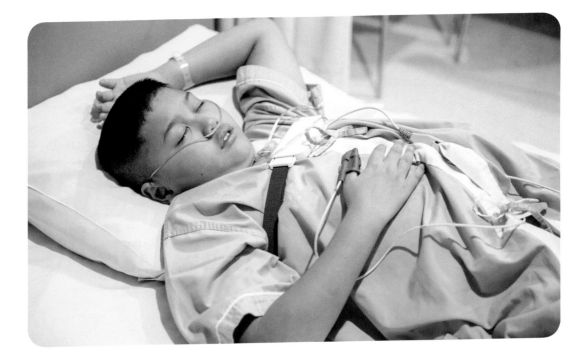

BEDWETTING

Bedwetting is a common problem among children, especially those under age six. Doctors don't know exactly what causes bedwetting or why it stops, but it often runs in families. Most of the time, bedwetting is not a sign of any medical or emotional problems.

Your child may feel embarrassed about wetting the bed and anxious about spending the night at a friend's house or at camp. Reassure him that bedwetting is a normal part of growing up and that it won't last

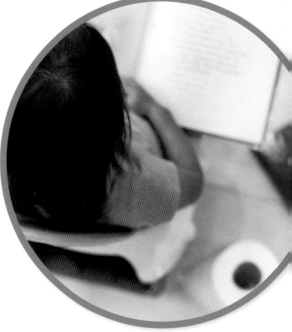

forever. It may comfort him to hear about other family members who struggled with bedwetting.

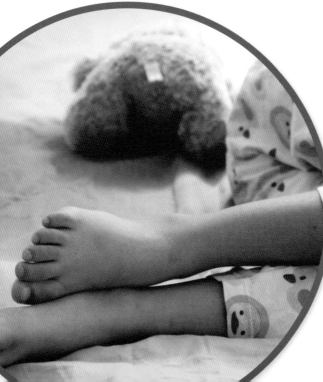

Have your child drink less at night, and avoid drinks that contain caffeine. Remind him to go to the bathroom one last time before bed. When your child wets the bed, don't yell or punish him. Have him help you change the sheets, but explain that this isn't punishment. Offer praise when your child has a dry night.

SUDDEN INFANT DEATH SYNDROME (SIDS)

Every year more than 2,000 infants in the United States die as a result of the terrifying yet unexplained phenomenon called sudden infant death syndrome (SIDS). Most SIDS deaths are associated with sleep, which is why it's sometimes called "crib death." In the U.S., SIDS is the leading cause of death among children between one month and one year of age, with most deaths occurring between two and four months. Although the cause is unknown, researchers have discovered some factors that might put infants at extra risk. They've also identified steps you can take to lower the risk. The most important step you can take is to always place your baby on his or her back to sleep—never on their stomach or side.

SIDS RISK FACTORS

- Baby sleeping on the stomach or side
- Using any soft or loose bedding, including quilts, heavy blankets, and bumper pads
- Baby sharing a sleep surface with parents, siblings, or pets
- Overheating or over-bundling baby
- Mother's smoking, drinking, or drug use during pregnancy and after birth
- Infant's exposure to secondhand smoke
- Poor prenatal care
- Prematurity or low birth weight
- Family history of SIDS
- Maternal age younger than 20
- Nonwhite infants are more likely to die of SIDS
- Slightly more boys die of SIDS than girls

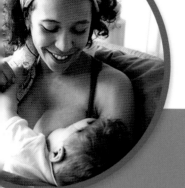

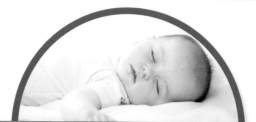

HOW TO REDUCE
THE RISK OF SIDS

- Get early and regular prenatal care.
- Don't smoke, drink, or use drugs while pregnant.
- Place your baby to sleep on his or her back, rather than on the stomach or side, every time for their first year of life.
- Keep the crib as bare as possible. Use a firm mattress with a fitted sheet and remove all loose bedding, pillows, stuffed toys, and other soft items from the crib.
- Don't use bumper pads in the crib.
- Have your baby sleep in your room, but alone in a crib or bassinet, for the first six months at least.
- Breastfeed your baby, if possible.
- Don't expose your baby to secondhand smoke after birth.
- Don't overheat your baby or cover your baby's head.
- Offer a pacifier (without a strap or string) at naptime and bedtime. If your baby rejects the pacifier, don't force it. If the pacifier falls out during sleep, don't replace it.
- Don't allow bed-sharing, even with siblings.
- Take your baby for their well-child appointments, including vaccinations.
- Don't use baby monitors and other products claiming to reduce the risk of SIDS.

Chapter 7: Sleep Medications

MEDICINES CAN PROFOUNDLY affect our sleep in both positive and negative ways. While sleep medicines can help with sleep for short periods of time, the lifestyle and sleep habit changes recommended in chapters 2–4 are the best long-term solutions for problems with insomnia.

In this chapter, we'll discuss the benefits and risks of using prescription or over-the-counter (OTC) medicines for sleep. Use of popular dietary and herbal supplements, including melatonin and valerian, are covered in chapter 8.

TYPES OF SLEEP AIDS

• **OVER-THE-COUNTER (OTC) SLEEP AIDS** are designed for short-term use to help you fall asleep. Most over-the-counter sleeping aids contain antihistamines, which are commonly used to treat allergies.

• **NATURAL SLEEP AIDS** include dietary and herbal supplements containing ingredients like melatonin, valerian, or chamomile. Natural sleep aids may come in herbal teas, pills, or ointments, and are available without a prescription. These are covered in the next chapter.

• **PRESCRIPTION DRUGS** target different parts of the brain to induce sleep. These drugs require a prescription from your doctor because they are stronger, have stronger side effects, and are more likely to become habit-forming.

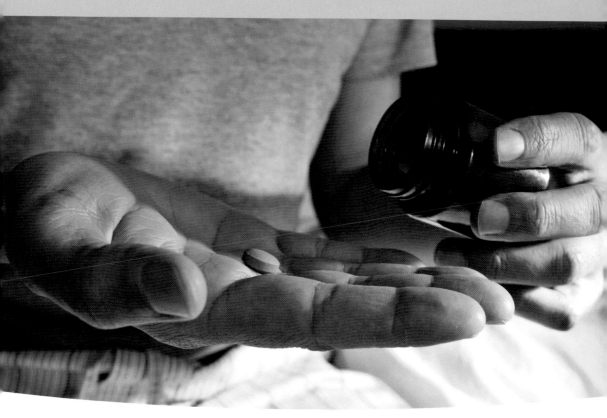

WHAT DRUGS CAN AND CAN'T DO

Sleep medication can't cure insomnia, regardless of how long you take it. Insomnia is a symptom of an underlying problem. Taking sleep medication over a long period of time actually masks the underlying problem instead of solving it.

Chronic use of sleep medication can create a physical and/or psychological dependence. It can also impair your ability to function the following day by causing lingering drowsiness or muddled thinking. Ironically, sleep medication can actually disrupt REM sleep and

WILL SLEEP MEDICATION HELP SNORING?

If you or your sleep partner snores, will a prescription or OTC sleep aid help stop the snoring by promoting deeper sleep? The answer: definitely not. In fact, it can create more problems. Sleep medications cause your muscles—including those in the throat area—to relax. As the muscles of the throat relax, a person who normally doesn't snore may actually start snoring. (Alcohol can have the same effect.)

Sleep medication can also further complicate breathing for the person who has severe apnea and put them into a potentially life-threatening situation. If you snore, and especially if you have already been diagnosed with sleep apnea, it's always recommended that you consult your doctor before taking any sleep aid.

On the positive side, sleep medications can be helpful to those who have short-term sleep disruptions caused by jet lag, shift-work rotations, or acute emotional difficulties such as divorce or loss of a loved one. To garner their benefits and limit their risks, it's important to take them only when they are truly needed, to find the right type of sleep medication for your needs, and to use them only for a brief period of time.

alter deep non-REM stages if used continually for more than two or three weeks.

OVER-THE-COUNTER (OTC) MEDICATIONS

Unlike the sleep aids that require a prescription from your doctor, over-the-counter (OTC) sleep aids can be purchased without a prescription in most supermarkets and drugstores. The active ingredient in most OTC sleep medications is antihistamine—the same antihistamine found in cold and allergy medications such as Benadryl. A natural side effect of antihistamines is drowsiness.

When drug companies found they could turn a drug side effect into a sleep-promoting benefit, they started marketing various OTC medications containing antihistamines as sleep aids.

While OTC sleep aids are generally not addictive, your body quickly builds up a tolerance to their sedative effects. As a result, they are less likely to help you fall asleep

REBOUND INSOMNIA

When you are physically dependent on some type of sleep medication and try to cut back or stop too quickly, you may experience a return of your insomnia. This is called rebound insomnia. Unfortunately, rebound insomnia leads many people to resume using their sleep medication when they actually need to reduce or discontinue use altogether. The only way to fight long-term insomnia is to find the source and treat it. Sleep medication should never be used as an acceptable long-term solution to insomnia.

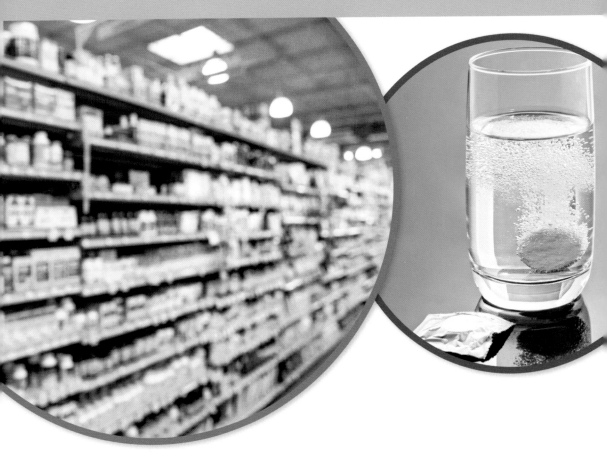

over time. And OTC sleep aids are not without side effects. OTC sleep aids may cause dry mouth, dizziness, constipation, hangover effects, and more. They can also cause memory problems in older adults.

An OTC sleep medication may help you survive a head cold, manage jet lag, or deal with some other minor and temporary sleep disruption, but it is not a solution to chronic insomnia. If you have ongoing sleep problems, consult your doctor. Be sure to inform your doctor of all medications (both prescription and OTC) and supplements you take.

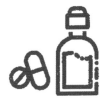

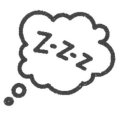

PRESCRIPTION MEDICATIONS

These medications require a prescription from your doctor because they are generally stronger and have more severe side effects than OTC medicines. Medications called hypnotics are the most commonly prescribed medicines for insomnia because they can help with sleep onset (the ability to fall asleep) and/or sleep maintenance (the ability to stay asleep). Most prescription sleep medications can become habit-forming and are only recommended for short-term use. Some of the most common prescription sleep medications are covered later in this chapter.

SLEEP AIDS AT A GLANCE

Drug type	How it works
Benzodiazepines	Slows brain activity by enhancing GABA activity
Non-benzodiazepines	Enhances GABA to slow brain activity
Orexin receptor antagonists	Inhibits chemical that increases alertness
Melatonin	Increases chemical responsible for sleep-wake cycle
Antidepressants	Sedates by altering serotonin and norepinephrine levels

BENZODIAZEPINES

Benzodiazepine receptor agonists (or benzodiazepines) enhance the action of GABA, a neurotransmitter that slows activity in the brain. These drugs were introduced in the 1960s to combat anxiety. They do promote sleep by depressing brain activity and inhibiting alertness, but they also reduce the duration of deep, non-REM sleep. Examples of benzodiazepines include diazepam (Valium), alprazolam (Xanax), lorazepam (Ativan), clonazepam (Klonopin), and chlordiazepoxide (Librium). Benzodiazepines are primarily used to treat anxiety disorders, though their sleep-inducing effects sometimes make them suitable as sleep aids. Their use for treating insomnia has declined since better drugs with fewer side effects and lower risk for dependency and abuse have been introduced.

NON-BENZODIAZEPINES

New prescription drugs called non-benzodiazepine receptor agonists (sometimes called non-benzodiazepine hypnotics or Z-drugs) for insomnia were introduced in the 1990s. Although structured differently than benzodiazepines, non-benzodiazepines work in a similar way. However, non-benzodiazepines tend to have fewer side effects and less impact on deep sleep. Common non-benzodiazepines include eszopiclone (Lunesta), zolpidem (Ambien), and zaleplon (Sonata). Because of proven effectiveness, reduced side effects, and less concern about addiction, non-benzodiazepines have become the most commonly prescribed medications for insomnia. Nevertheless, these drugs are not without risks. Non-benzodiazepines can cause side effects such as memory loss, next-day impairment and fatigue, and rare cases of driving, talking on the phone, eating, or having sex while partially asleep with no memory afterward.

By blocking orexin, these drugs may help promote sleep. Suvorexant (brand name Belsomra) is one FDA-approved orexin receptor antagonist.

OREXIN RECEPTOR ANTAGONISTS

The most recent class of insomnia drugs is orexin receptor antagonists. They work by inhibiting the activity of the chemical orexin in the brain. Orexin (also called hypocretin) is a neuropeptide that regulates wakefulness, arousal, and hunger.

MELATONIN

Melatonin is a hormone produced in the pineal gland that regulates the circadian cycle of sleep and wakefulness. Levels of melatonin naturally rise at night, inducing sleepiness. Melatonin has relatively few side effects and is not known to cause dependence. But melatonin is less effective than other sleep aids. Ramelteon (brand name Rozerem) is a common prescription melatonin. Melatonin is also available as an over-the-counter supplement, but it may be even less effective than prescription melatonin. Melatonin supplements are covered in more detail in chapter 8.

ANTIDEPRESSANTS

For people struggling with both insomnia and depression, certain antidepressant medications can help treat the mood disorder and restore restful sleep. Certain antidepressants are known to have a fairly strong sedating effect early on in treatment, even in people who don't suffer from depression. This initial sedating effect generally wears off, however, as the body adjusts to the drug. Some doctors, therefore, may prescribe one of these sedating antidepressants for short-term treatment of insomnia in people who don't have depression. Antidepressants prescribed for sleep include doxepin (Adapin, Sinequan, Silenor, Zonalon), trazodone (Oleptro), mirtazapine (Remeron), and amitriptyline (Elavil, Endep). As with all medications, antidepressants can cause side effects. Talk with your doctor if you think an antidepressant may be appropriate for you.

COMMON PRESCRIPTION SLEEP DRUGS

ZALEPLON (Sonata)

Zaleplon (brand name Sonata) is a sedative-hypnotic used to treat short-term insomnia in patients that have difficulty falling asleep. Zaleplon does not help you stay asleep longer or reduce the number of times you wake up during the night. Sonata is available in 5- and 10-milligram capsules. It is usually taken at bedtime or after trying unsuccessfully to fall asleep. Zaleplon can be habit-forming.

Don't take zaleplon with or shortly after a heavy, high-fat meal. Side effects may include drowsiness, dizziness, numbness or tingling at the extremities, poor coordination, headache, loss of appetite, eye pain and vision problems, sensitivity to noise and smell, and painful menstrual periods. Some people have reported getting out of bed while not fully awake and driving a car, preparing and eating food, talking on the phone, having sex, or sleepwalking after taking zaleplon.

. . . .

ZOLPIDEM (Ambien, Ambien CR, Edluar, Intermezzo)

Zolpidem is a sedative-hypnotic that is used to treat short-term insomnia in people who having difficulty falling asleep or staying asleep. Zolpidem is available as a tablet (brand name Ambien), an extended-

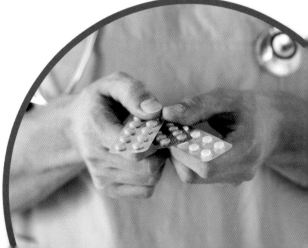

release tablet (Ambien CR), a sublingual tablet (Edluar and Intermezzo) to place under the tongue, and an oral spray (Zolpimist). Plan to go to bed immediately after taking zolpidem tablets, extended-release tablets, Edluar sublingual tablets, or oral spray and to stay in bed for seven to eight hours. The Intermezzo sublingual tablets are designed to help people who wake up in the middle of the night return to sleep. Take Intermezzo only when you can remain in bed for at least four more hours.

Zolpidem can be habit-forming and should only be taken for short periods of time. Side effects may include drowsiness, dizziness, diarrhea, headache, grogginess or drugged feeling, decreased motor coordination, and unusual dreams. After taking zolpidem, you may get out of bed and drive a car, sleepwalk, have sex, eat food, or make phone calls while partially asleep. Next-day impairment is an issue with zolpidem and other sleep medications like it. Avoid driving a car or performing other activities for which you must be fully alert the morning after taking zolpidem. You may be impaired even if you feel fully awake.

ESZOPICLONE (Lunesta)

Eszopiclone (brand name Lunesta) is a hypnotic used to treat insomnia in people who have difficulty falling asleep and staying asleep. Eszopiclone is longer lasting than some other sleep medications and thus helps maintain sleep longer. It is also less likely to cause dependence and is approved for long-term use. Eszopiclone is available in 1-, 2-, and 3-milligram tablets.

Don't take eszopiclone with or shortly after a meal—especially a heavy, high-fat meal. Side effects of eszopiclone may include drowsiness, dizziness, unpleasant taste or dry mouth, headache, loss of coordination, and cold symptoms. Don't drive a car or perform other dangerous activities the day after taking eszopiclone until you feel fully awake. Driving a car, sleepwalking, having sex, eating, and making phone calls while partially asleep have been reported with eszopiclone.

RAMELTEON (Rozerem)

Ramelteon (brand name Rozerem) is used to treat sleep-onset insomnia (difficulty falling asleep). Ramelteon belongs to a class of medications called melatonin receptor agonists. Melatonin is a hormone produced in the pineal gland that helps regulate sleep. Like zaleplon (Sonata), zolpidem (Ambien), and eszopiclone (Lunesta), ramelteon may cause next-day impairment and cases of performing activities such as driving, walking, talking, eating, and having sex while partially asleep have been reported. But unlike most other prescription sleep medications, ramelteon has not been shown to cause dependency. Ramelteon is available in 8-milligram tablets. Take ramelteon within 30 minutes of going to bed, not sooner. Only take ramelteon if you are able to stay asleep for at least seven to eight hours before becoming active.

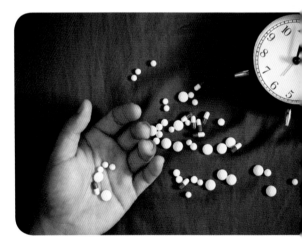

Don't take ramelteon with or right after a meal. Common side effects include drowsiness and dizziness. Don't take ramelteon if you take the antidepressant fluvoxamine (Luvox), which is primarily used to treat obsessive-compulsive disorder (OCD).

COMMON PRESCRIPTION SLEEP AIDS

Generic Name	Brand Name	Dosage(s)	Helps you fall asleep	Helps you stay asleep	Can lead to dependence
Benzodiazepines					
Triazolam	Halcion	0.125, 0.25 mg tablets	Yes	No	Yes
Temaze-pam	Restoril	7.5, 15, 22.5, 30 mg tablets	Yes	Yes	Yes
Estazolam	ProSom	1, 2 mg tablets	Yes	Yes	Yes
Non-benzodiazepines					
Eszopi-clone	Lunesta	1, 2, 3 mg tablets	Yes	Yes	Yes
Zaleplon	Sonata	5, 10 mg capsules	Yes	No	Yes
Zolpidem	Ambien	5, 10 mg tablets	Yes	No	Yes
Zolpidem extended release	Ambien CR	6.25, 12.5 mg tablets	Yes	Yes	Yes
Zolpidem	Edluar	5, 10 mg sublingual tablets	Yes	No	Yes
Zolpidem	Inter-mezzo	1.75, 3.5 mg sublingual tablets	Yes	No	Yes
Zolpidem	Zolpi-mist	5 mg spray	Yes	No	Yes

Generic Name	Brand Name	Dosage(s)	Helps you fall asleep	Helps you stay asleep	Can lead to dependence
Melatonin					
Ramelteon	Rozerem	8 mg tablets	Yes	No	Yes
Orexin receptor antagonist					
Suvorexant	Bel-somra	10 mg tablets	Yes	Yes	Yes
Antidepressant					
Doxepin	Silenor	3, 6 mg tablets	No	Yes	No

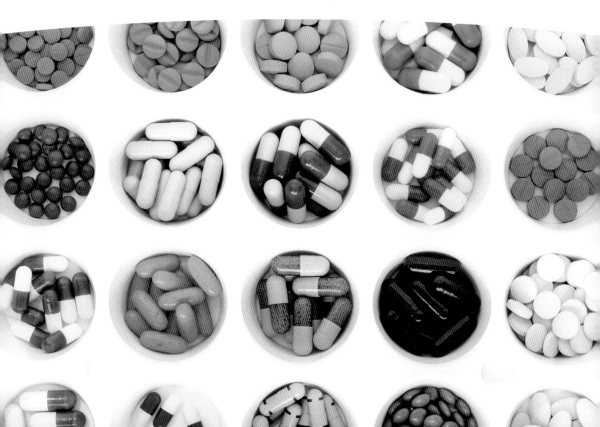

USING SLEEP MEDICATION WISELY

Here are some guidelines on how to use sleep medication wisely.

• Talk to your doctor before you start taking any sleep medications. To avoid potentially serious interactions, be sure to inform all of your health care providers of all prescription and over-the-counter medicines, supplements, and herbal remedies you're taking.

• Don't drink alcohol with any sleep medication. Alcohol worsens the sedating effects of sleep medication. Mixing the two could have deadly results.

• Use the smallest possible dose of any sleep medication. Don't increase the recommended or prescribed dose without your doctor's approval.

• Take your sleep medication on an empty stomach. This will allow it to be absorbed more quickly and work faster. Avoid taking sleep medication at the same time you take antacids, which slow the stomach's action.

• Don't take your sleep medication until you're ready to go to bed. You shouldn't be doing any activities that require concentration or are stimulating during this time. The only thing you should be doing after taking sleep medication is preparing to sleep.

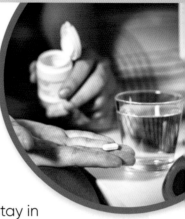

• Only take your sleep medication when you can get a full night's sleep (at least seven to eight hours). A few short-acting medications, such as Intermezzo, are intended for middle of the night awakenings, so you may take them when you can stay in bed for at least four more hours.

• Don't use sleep medication for more than two or three weeks. Most prescription sleep aids for insomnia are only approved for use up to one month.

• Try to limit your use of sleep medication to no more than three nights per week. Following this rule can help ensure that you don't build up a tolerance to the medication. You'll therefore be more likely to get the full benefit from the recommended dose of the drug without having to take larger and larger doses.

• Treat the primary problem first. If your insomnia is related to depression, seek treatment for the depression first. If you can't sleep because you are experiencing another symptom such as pain, ask for a pain reliever or for treatment that will remedy the cause of the pain instead of for a sleeping pill.

• Search for the underlying cause of your insomnia. Remember, insomnia is a symptom. The goal of using sleep medication is to get you through a short-term period of sleeplessness. Examine the possible sources of your insomnia such as stress, irregular bedtimes, and caffeine intake. If you don't address the source of your insomnia, you unnecessarily tempt yourself to depend on sleep medications.

• Before taking sleep medication, tell your doctor if you are pregnant, plan to become pregnant, or are breastfeeding.

• Sleep medication can impair your ability to drive and perform other activities for which you need to be fully alert the next day. Your ability to drive may be impaired the day after taking zolpidem even if you feel fully awake.

• Some people taking prescription sleep medication drove their cars, ate food, had sex, made phone calls, were sleepwalking, or were involved in other activities while not fully awake. You have a higher chance for doing this if you drink alcohol or take other medicines that make you sleepy with your sleep medication.

• Your sleep problems should improve within seven to ten days after starting your sleep medication. If your sleep problems don't improve or get worse within this time, call your doctor.

• Don't suddenly stop taking prescription medication without talking to your doctor. You may have symptoms of withdrawal. Your doctor will probably decrease your dose gradually instead.

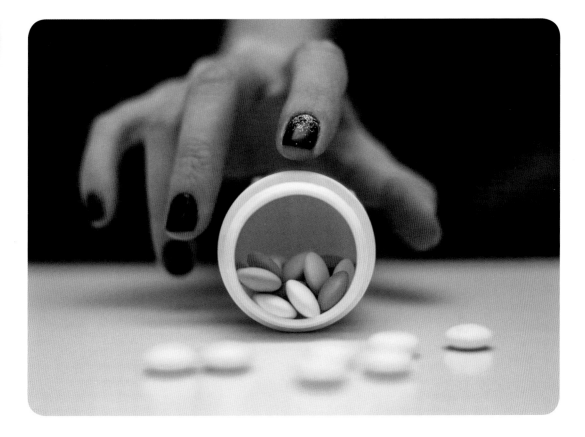

KICKING THE PILL HABIT

Because over half of the American population is struggling with sleep problems—whether due to poor lifestyle choices or severe sleep disorders—many are turning to sleep medications for help. And sizable numbers are using these medications every night for weeks, months, even years on end. Most don't know they are actually making their sleep problems worse.

But say that you recognize that your chronic use of sleep aids is working against you, and you want to escape the sleeping pill trap. How do you do it?

• Your first step is to talk with your physician. Anytime you've been using sleep medication for an extended amount of time, you don't want to just stop "cold turkey." Your doctor may develop a specific plan for you to gradually reduce the dosage until you can stop entirely. Tell your doctor about your goals to stop using the sleep medication.

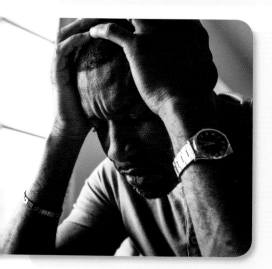

• Don't consider cutting back on medication if your life is particularly hectic or stressful. Wait for some stability or for the immediate crises to pass, if possible. You'll need at least four weeks to completely wean yourself from most sleep medications.

• If you find your anxiety increases as your medication is reduced, add some relaxation techniques into your bed-time ritual. These might include listening to soothing music, practicing visualization, or using breathing exercises (see chapter 3 for more suggestions). These techniques can also be used as part of a "sleepless plan," for those inevitable nights when you won't be able to sleep as well as you'd like.

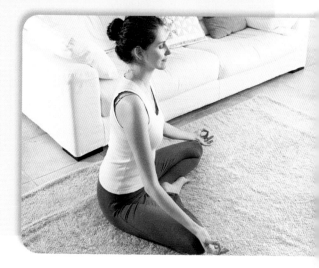

Chapter 8: Complementary Health Approaches for Sleep

MANY PEOPLE VIEW HEALTH practices that are outside conventional mainstream medicine with skepticism. They bring to mind images of witch doctors, tonic peddlers, and those hawking "miracle" supplements and gadgets on late-night TV ads. We are justified in being skeptical of any products that promise cures and carry no proof of effectiveness. Such scams, unfortunately, can mask the fact that there are a few non-mainstream approaches that may help you manage your health and your sleep.

In this chapter, we'll examine some of the many ways you can improve your sleep with complementary health approaches.

These include mind and body practices such as acupuncture, massage therapy, yoga, and meditation, as well as natural products such as herbs and other botanicals, vitamins and minerals, and dietary supplements. None of these approaches are intended to replace conventional medical treatment for serious sleep disorders or insomnia that causes severe daytime fatigue; such conditions require medical intervention. But some of the complementary health approaches covered here may work in concert with conventional medical treatment and lifestyle changes to improve your overall sleep.

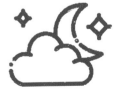
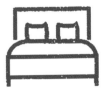

COMPLEMENTARY VS. ALTERNATIVE MEDICINE

More than 30 percent of Americans report using health care approaches that are not typically part of conventional mainstream medicine. When describing these approaches, people often use the terms "complementary" and "alternative" interchangeably, but they refer to different things:

• **Complementary medicine is used** *in addition to* **conventional medicine.**
• **Alternative medicine is used** *instead of* **conventional medicine.**

Many doctors and health care facilities are combining complementary medicine with conventional mainstream medicine, spawning the term "integrative medicine."

COMPLEMENTARY HEALTH PRODUCTS AND PRACTICES

• **Mind and body practices** include a wide variety of procedures and techniques, such as acupuncture, massage therapy, chiropractic and osteopathic manipulation, yoga, tai chi, qi gong, meditation, hypnotherapy, and relaxation techniques.

• **Natural products** include vitamins, minerals, herbs and other botanicals, probiotics, amino acids, and other dietary supplements.

• **Other complementary health approaches**—such as the practices of traditional healers, Ayurvedic medicine, traditional Chinese medicine, homeopathy, naturopathy, and functional medicine—may not neatly fit into either of these groups.

ACUPUNCTURE AND ACUPRESSURE

Acupuncture dates back thousands of years and is rooted in Eastern healing practices. It's based on a concept that all disease, including sleep problems, is the result of an imbalance of subtle energy moving throughout the body. This energy moves along 14 pathways in the body called meridians. Through the ages, practitioners have identified and charted these meridians. Treatment by an acupuncturist involves inserting very fine needles at various points along these meridians to increase, decrease, or balance the energy flow.

In the Western scientific community, there is a great deal of skepticism about the use of acupuncture, mainly because there have not been a lot of well-designed, well-controlled studies proving its effectiveness. The National Institutes of Health, however, has stated that there is enough evidence to indicate that acupuncture can be helpful in controlling nausea and certain types of pain. Acupuncture has also been suggested—and in the East, used—as a remedy for insomnia, although scientific proof of this particular benefit is lacking. Still, acupuncture might be worth a try, especially for people suffering from chronic pain that affects their ability to get enough restful sleep.

Most people have heard about someone who has been helped by acupuncture but are reluctant to try it themselves because they fear having needles inserted into their body. But the consensus of most people who have used acupuncture is that the procedure causes little or no discomfort, and many swear by the benefits they've received. Side effects from acupuncture are also rare and appear to result mostly from treatment by unqualified practitioners.

If you decide to try acupuncture for your sleep problems, seek out a licensed practitioner, if your state governs this profession, or one certified by the National Commission for the Certification of Acupuncturists. In addition, check to be sure the acupuncturist uses sterile, disposable needles, to decrease any risk of transmission of blood-borne infectious organisms.

A close cousin of acupuncture is acupressure. Acupressure relies on the same meridian points as acupuncture, but finger pressure, rather than a needle, is used to stimulate points along the meridians to increase, decrease, or balance the energy running through the body.

ACUPRESSURE SELF-HELP

There are professional practitioners of acupressure, but this is one technique you can try on your own as well. To combat insomnia, try massaging the following pressure points:

• The fleshy tissue between your big toe and second toe. Feel for the tenderest spot, and massage for about two minutes.

• The crease of your wrist. With your palm facing up, follow the inside edge of your hand down from the pinky to the crease at the wrist, just under the bone. Massage and press firmly for two to three minutes.

• The area below the inner anklebone. Put your thumb on your inner anklebone (the rounded bone that sticks out just above the inner side of your foot). Then slide your thumb down about a finger's width. Massage and apply pressure to this fleshy area for two to three minutes.

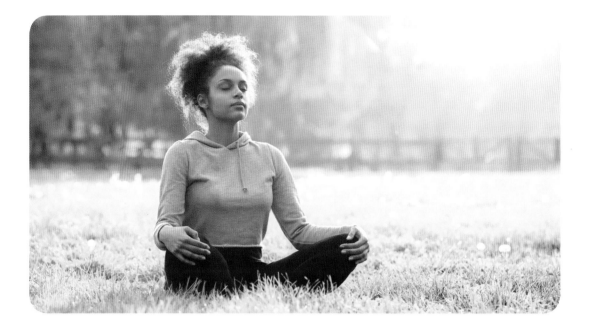

MINDFULNESS AND MEDITATION

Ever had a night, or a string of nights, when you couldn't sleep because of troublesome thoughts or worries? Of course, we all have. Meditation is an excellent way to control those thoughts and is a safe and simple way to balance your physical, emotional, and mental states. Mindfulness meditation can help you pull your mind away from concerns about the past or future and focus on the present moment.

Meditation is not so much an emptying of the mind as it is a calming of the mind. One of the first things people realize when they begin meditating is how fast and furious their thoughts bombard them when they try to be still.

One novice meditator found this to be the case when he signed up for a local class on meditation. On the first night of instruction, he was told to lie on the floor and simply pay attention to his breathing for ten minutes. He thought to himself, "That's it? That'll be easy." He closed his eyes and, within seconds, it was like someone had pushed the play button on his mental DVR. Work hassles, bills, errands, plots from TV programs, and more ran through his mind like an old silent film set on fast-forward. By the time the ten minutes had elapsed, he felt more tense than when he started. But the experience gave him a clue about why he was having so much trouble falling asleep at night and why he felt so uptight and hurried all the time. After several weeks of participating in the class and practicing what he learned, he was gradually able to start roping in some of his worrisome thoughts and found that he could fall asleep much easier when he slipped into bed at night.

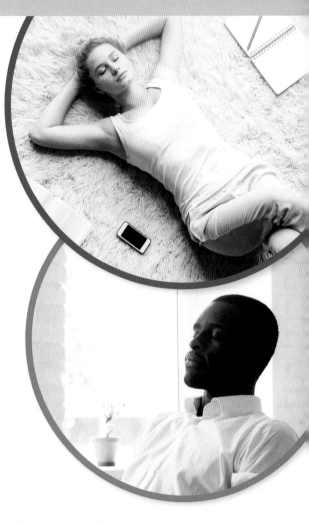

During meditation, the pulse rate slows, blood pressure falls, blood supply to the arms and legs increases, levels of stress hormones drop, and brain waves resemble a state of relaxation found in the early stages of sleep. These are all physical changes that can be brought about by learning to clear your mind of clutter and focus your thoughts. You can use meditation to clear and refresh your mind during the day or help you relax at night in preparation for sleep.

Although meditation sounds easy, it takes some practice to be most effective. Perhaps the hardest part is being able to block out intruding thoughts that threaten the peacefulness you seek. But if you practice every day, it will become easier, and you're likely to find that you look forward to these respites from your busy life. You're also likely to discover that sleep comes much more easily to a quiet, relaxed mind.

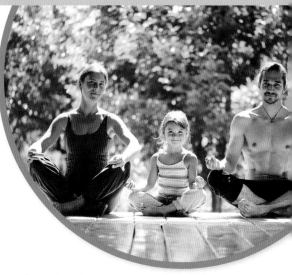

Being mindful means being completely present to the feelings, sensations, and experiences of the moment. It means putting away watches and phones and devices and tuning into nature or the sound of your own breath. It means having no sense of worry, need, fear, demand, or expectation of what should be and instead allowing life to unfold as is. Mindfulness requires no equipment or membership.

You only need:

- A quiet place free from interruptions

- Music, a guided meditation, or pure silence

- The ability to sit still for at least ten minutes

- To experience what is, without resistance

- Patience to focus and center your breathing

- The desire to live a more balanced, harmonious life

A SIMPLE MEDITATION EXERCISE

Despite a popular myth, you don't need to contort your body into a cross-legged lotus position to meditate. A sitting or lying position will do just fine. (If you choose a sitting position, keep your spine straight but your shoulders relaxed.) It also helps to have a quiet place where you won't be distracted or disturbed. Once you're situated, close your eyes and breathe slowly, feeling the air enter your lungs. Next, exhale slowly, feeling the air leave your body. Keep the focus on your breathing. If your mind wanders off, gently bring your focus back to your breathing. You want your attention to remain on your breathing to keep you in the present moment. This way you won't be distracted by past or future events that may carry your mind away and possibly bring anxiety.

Practice this for 15 minutes each day. It can be especially helpful right before bed if you notice your mind is racing.

MINDFULNESS-BASED STRESS REDUCTION

A preliminary study found that mindfulness-based stress reduction (MBSR), a type of meditation, was as effective as a prescription drug in a small group of people with insomnia. Mindfulness-based stress reduction is a program that combines mindfulness meditation, body scanning, and yoga. Classes and programs typically focus on teaching non-judgmental mind and body awareness to reduce the physiological effects of stress, pain, or illness.

USE RELAXATION TECHNIQUES

Relaxation techniques are one of the most promising complementary health approaches for insomnia. Evidence shows that using relaxation techniques before bedtime can be part of a successful strategy to improve sleep habits. Other components discussed in chapters 2–4 include maintaining a consistent sleep schedule; avoiding caffeine, alcohol, heavy meals, and strenuous exercise too close to bedtime; and sleeping in a quiet, cool, and dark room.

See chapter 3 (pages 57–59) for the active relaxation techniques of progressive muscle relaxation, abdominal breathing, and visualization. Practicing these relaxation techniques is an excellent way to quiet your body and mind before bed.

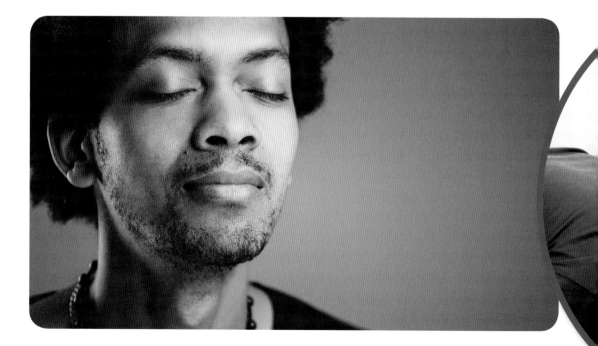

MASSAGE

Massage is one of several hands-on strategies known collectively as bodywork. And if you've ever had a good, thorough massage, you know the feeling of being "worked over." But you also know how relaxing it can be.

The benefits of massage are many. It is regularly used in sports clinics and rehabilitation centers to loosen or soothe sore, aching muscles. Massage also helps to reduce stress, improve circulation, release tension, lower heart rate and blood pressure, and possibly even strengthen the immune system. These relaxing effects may therefore make massage a helpful aid in restoring restful sleep. Massage may be especially beneficial in treating sleeping problems that stem from stress, migraine headache, pain, and muscle and joint stiffness.

You might want to spring for a massage from a professional. One session may be all it takes to get you hooked. If you do opt for a professional massage, be sure to tell the practitioner if you have any particular illness or injury that they should be aware of, such as arthritis or fibromyalgia.

One of the good things about massage, of course, is that you don't have to visit a professional to capture its benefits. You can ask your partner, friend, or family member for a soothing rubdown. You can also give yourself a mini massage, focusing on the muscle groups that are within reach. Using small, circular movements with

HOMEMADE MASSAGE OIL

Oil allows your hands to move freely over the body during massage. While a variety of massage oils are on the market, you can also make your own. Choose a vegetable-based oil that has little or no scent of its own. Almond oil is a good choice because it is light and odorless. Avoid olive oil, which is too heavy and pungent. Then, to enhance the experience, you can add a few drops of an aromatic essential oil, such as lavender or chamomile, both of which tend to have a relaxing effect.

your fingers and hands, you can massage your scalp, forehead, face, neck and upper shoulders, lower back, arms, legs, and feet. There are also a variety of massaging devices available in various price ranges that can help extend your reach or provide soothing heat as well as relaxing vibrations.

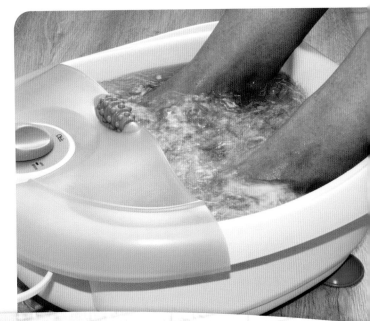

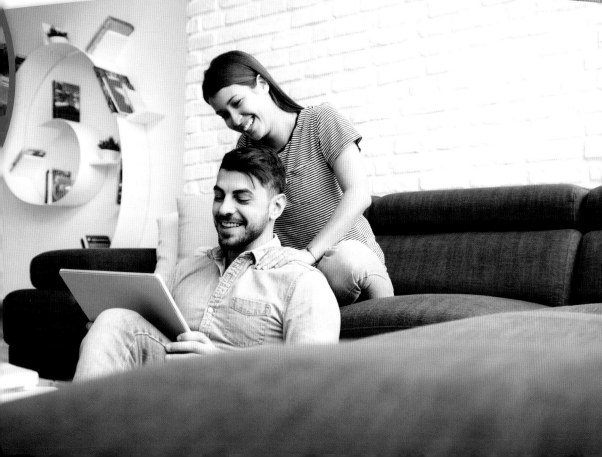

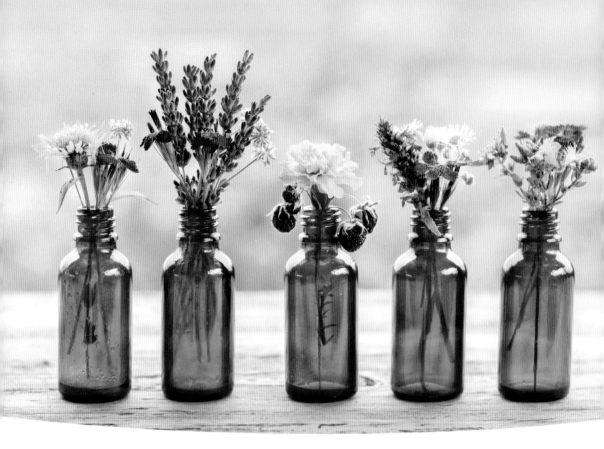

AROMATHERAPY

Aromatherapy is the therapeutic use of essential oils to comfort and heal. In aromatherapy, the essential oils are used topically rather than taken internally. The essential oils are said to stimulate an area of the brain known as the limbic system that controls mood and emotion. Solid scientific backing for aromatherapy is lacking, but there's no doubt that many people find it a soothing complement to other self-help measures to ease tension, promote relaxation, and aid in sleep as part of their bedtime preparations. So you may want to give it a try.

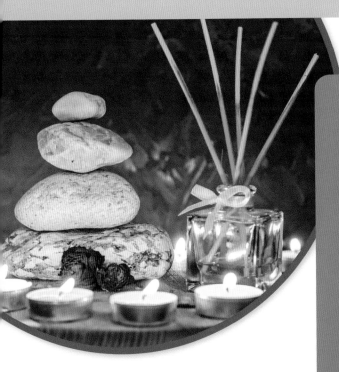

CALMING ESSENTIAL OILS

- Bergamot
- Chamomile
- Clary sage
- Lavender
- Lemon balm
- Orange
- Rose
- Sandalwood
- Sweet marjoram
- Ylang-ylang

To help restore restful sleep, you can try using essential oils individually or in combination. The essential oils are generally available at health food stores, although these days many drugstores also carry a variety of the oils. The most commonly recommended oil for promoting sleep is lavender, but there are several others that may have a calming effect (see the sidebar on the right).

Try adding a few drops of essential oil to warm water for a relaxing bath or footbath, or spritz the oil onto a handkerchief or small pillow. You can also apply a few drops to a heat diffuser near your bed to

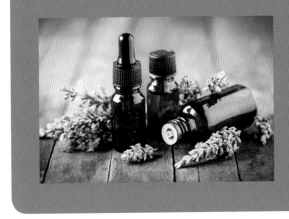

spread the scent through the room or use a specially made ring that can be placed on the lightbulb of a bedside lamp; the heat of the bulb diffuses the scent.

You might also want to try combining the relaxing benefits of aromatherapy and massage by creating your own scented massage oil. Dilute one to three drops of essential oil per teaspoon of an unscented carrier oil, such as almond or grape-seed oil. (Do not apply undiluted essential oil directly to your skin.) Since some people are more sensitive to the oils than others, start with the smallest amount, and experiment until you find the combination that works best for you.

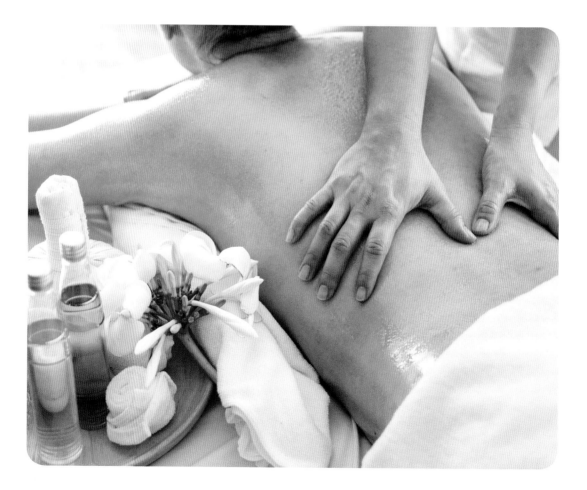

MAKE A SCENTED SLEEP PILLOW

Having a pleasant scent filling your nostrils when you get into bed may help you drift off to dreamland. A scented pillow is one way to create this effect. To make a scented pillow, you can, of course, spray a bit of essential oil onto your regular pillow. But you can also make an herb-filled sleep pillow by combining aromatic herbs and sewing them into a small piece of soft fabric. You'll want the pillow to be small and flat, so you can slip it into your regular pillowcase, on top of your regular pillow. Here's a sweet but potent mixture for an herbal pillow:

- 4 parts dried lavender leaves
- 2 parts dried hops
- 2 parts dried rose petals
- 1 part dried chamomile
- 1 part dried lemon balm

The herbs eventually lose their scent and should be replaced after about 9 to 12 months.

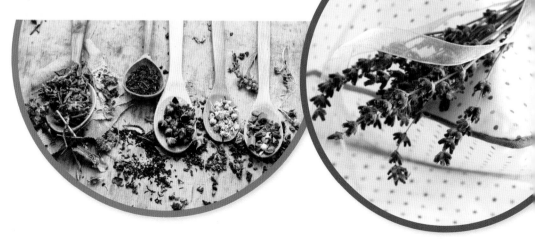

BIOFEEDBACK

Stress can put a major dent in your ability to sleep. Since no one can completely escape stress, the best way to keep it from stealing your shut-eye is to learn to manage your response to it. Toward that end, you may want to give a technique called biofeedback a try.

Biofeedback training can help you learn to consciously control certain physical responses to stress. It begins with the use of a simple electronic device that monitors your heart rate, breathing, blood pressure, and/or muscle tension through electrodes that are placed on your skin. These electrodes give "feedback" about what your body is doing under certain conditions. You can then use this feedback to retrain your responses.

For instance, when you are in a stressful situation—or even when you are just thinking about one—your heart rate tends to speed up, your breathing quickens, your blood pressure increases, and your muscles tense up. Conversely, by shifting your thoughts to calming scenes or situations or by consciously taking slow, deep breaths, you can slow your heart rate, lower your blood pressure, and ease muscle tension. The biofeedback machine makes these reactions easier to recognize. For example, the machine may be set to beep at every heartbeat, so you can hear when your heart is racing or when it's slowing. The

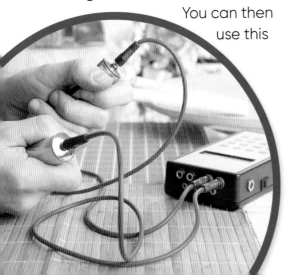

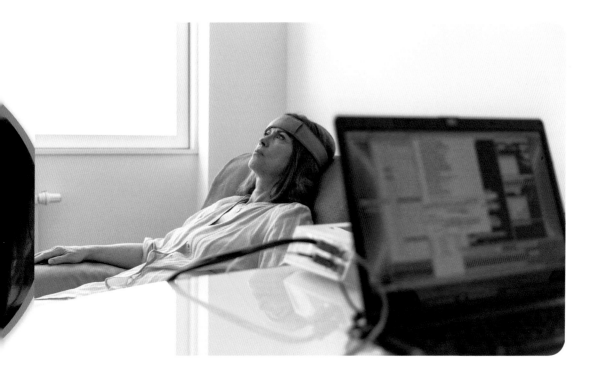

combination of this feedback with training in relaxation techniques, such as visualization, meditation, or even simple breathing exercises, can thus help you to notice when stress is negatively affecting your body and actively take steps to reverse those effects. With practice, you become better able to recognize stress responses so that eventually you no longer need the biofeedback machine. In this way, biofeedback can help individuals whose sleep problems stem from poor stress management, anxiety, or obsessive thoughts.

Most people who decide to try biofeedback visit a clinic where a trained professional in biofeedback can guide them through the process. If you take this route, look for a biofeedback practitioner who is certified by the Biofeedback Certification Institute of America. The option of purchasing inexpensive biofeedback equipment to use on your own is also available. These home units typically come with detailed instructions for proper use.

SELF-HYPNOSIS

Stage acts or television programs you've seen might give you the impression that hypnosis is about losing control. But actually, it is about gaining control. A person who is truly hypnotized is in a deep state of relaxation and is fully aware of what is going on around them. For this very reason, self-hypnosis may prove helpful in relieving sleep problems associated with stress. It provides a tool that you can use to induce a deep state of relaxation whenever you want to.

There are many methods of self-hypnosis. Here's one that's fairly easy. Choose a positive statement that expresses a desire. For instance, "Each breath makes me feel more relaxed." Once you have the statement in mind, lie down and take three slow, deep breaths. Close your eyes and, starting at your head, begin using your affirmation statement on different parts of your body. "Each breath makes my forehead more relaxed." As you breathe, imagine releasing any tension in that part of your body when you exhale. Move to the next part: "Each breath makes my jaw more relaxed." Continue using the same affirmative statement with various parts of your body until you finish with your toes. Continue regular, slow, deep breaths throughout.

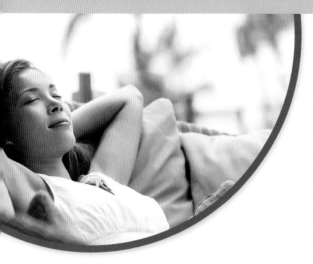

It could be indoors or outdoors, as long as it is peaceful and inviting to you. Once there, repeat your affirmation statement three times. Stay and enjoy the place for as long as you like. When you feel ready to leave, say goodbye to your special place. Then, before opening your eyes, tell yourself that you will slowly count from one to three and that by the time you reach three and open your eyes, you will feel fully relaxed and ready to enjoy peaceful sleep.

Then count backward from 100 to 95 and immediately imagine yourself being taken to a serene setting that you would like to visit.

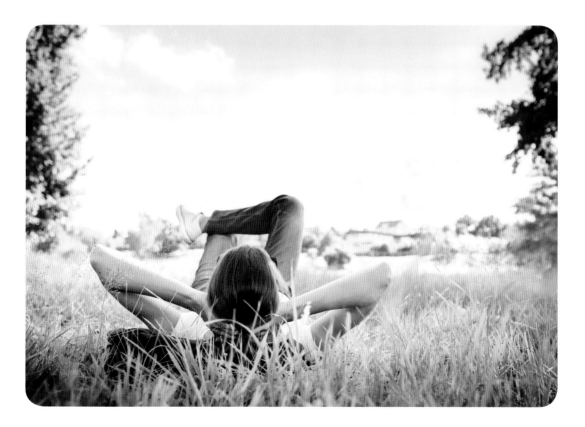

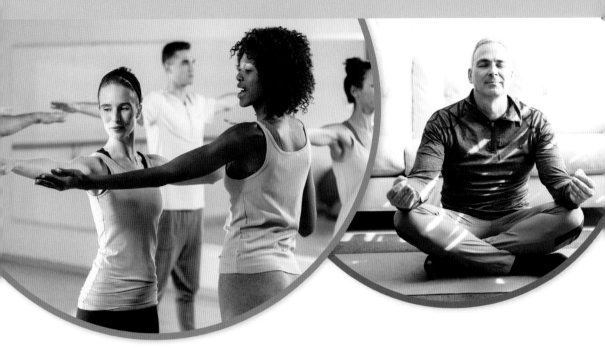

YOGA

Yoga, from India, is one of the world's oldest health practices. Although often associated with Eastern religions and practices, more and more Westerners are adopting it for its numerous benefits. The most notable of these are increased circulation, better flexibility of muscles and joints, relaxation, and improved sleep.

Yoga is based on the principle that the mind, body, and spirit work in unison. If the body is sick, it affects the mind and spirit. If the mind is chronically restless and agitated, the health of the body and spirit will be affected. And if the spirit is depleted, the mind and body will suffer. There are many forms of yoga, many of which use various poses that incorporate stretching and breathing exercises to integrate mind, body, and spirit. (Don't worry: You don't have to lay on a bed of nails or twist your body into a pretzel shape to achieve yoga's benefits.)

Yoga can help with sleep problems by loosening tight muscles, releasing tension, and putting you into a deep state of relaxation. But it's a type of relaxation that requires fixed attention to work well. The breathing and stretching exercises are designed to slow down your racing thoughts and pull you into the present moment. The practice of yoga helps stem the flow of stress hormones that your body produces when you are under stress. Indeed, when your body, mind, and spirit are connected and relaxed, you are more resilient to stress. You will also undoubtedly sleep better.

Try one of these exercises before getting into bed to enhance relaxation.

• Lie on the floor or a bed with your arms near your sides and your legs slightly parted. Relax your entire body by letting it sink into the floor or bed. Breathe in slowly through your nose, and pull the air deeply into your lungs until you feel your abdomen rise. Slowly exhale. Be attentive to how your body feels as you breathe in and out. Repeat with as many breaths as you need to feel calm.

• Sitting comfortably in a straight-backed chair, with your back supported and legs uncrossed, practice the same breathing technique mentioned in the previous exercise. After two or three deep breaths, raise your hands above your head and stretch as if you were trying to touch the ceiling. Continue breathing while you stretch. Be attentive to how your body and your mind feel as you breathe. Repeat until you feel more relaxed and ready to sleep.

• Standing, with your feet shoulder-width apart, inhale deeply, clasp your hands together and raise them above your head, and gently rise up on your toes. Stretch your whole body upward. Exhale slowly as you bring your arms back down to your sides and lower your heels to the floor. Repeat one or two more times.

DO A SIMPLE QI GONG EXERCISE

The first step in performing a qi gong exercise is to locate the Dantian, a major energy center in the body near the solar plexus. The point is located below the naval at a distance equal to the width of four fingers. The acupuncture point located there is called "Gate to the Original Qi," and the Dantian is located inside the abdomen about a third of the distance between that point and the spine. This is the focus of meditation during qi gong exercises.

While performing qi gong, it's most important to relax and be calm. Sitting on the floor cross-legged or with legs extended, shoulders relaxed and hands facing down in your lap, meditate on the Dantian as you inhale normally. Continue focusing on your Dantian while you exhale normally, then slowly lean forward and slide your hands out in front of you on the floor. You should be fully stretched out by the end of the exhale, not forcing either the stretch or the breathing. Gradually sit up to the original position as you inhale, continuing your meditation on the energy center. Repeat for a few minutes, then discontinue the focused meditation and sit still with your eyes closed, breathing normally.

After a qi gong session, people typically feel energized and relaxed, ready to deal with the stresses of the world in a calm and grounded manner.

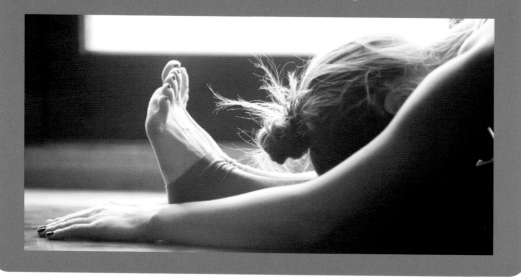

MELATONIN AND RELATED SUPPLEMENTS

Melatonin is a hormone produced by the pineal gland. It plays an important role in sleep. The production and release of melatonin is related to the time of day, rising at night and falling in the morning. Darkness signals the body to make melatonin while light blocks melatonin production. Current evidence suggests that melatonin supplements may be useful in treating several sleep disorders, such as delayed sleep phase disorder, insomnia, jet lag, and sleep problems related to shift work.

DELAYED SLEEP PHASE DISORDER

Melatonin has been used as a tool to treat delayed sleep phase disorder (a disruption of the body's biological clock). Adolescents and adults with this disorder generally fall asleep well after midnight and have trouble waking up in the morning. When used in combination with reduced evening light and behavioral changes, melatonin supplements may help even out sleep cycles. The American Academy of Sleep Medicine supports timed melatonin supplementation for delayed sleep phase disorder.

SHIFT WORK

About two million Americans who work afternoon to nighttime or nighttime to early morning hours are affected by shift work disorder. Because their work schedules are at odds with powerful sleep-regulating cues like sunlight, night shift workers often feel drowsy at work, and have difficulty falling or staying asleep during the daylight hours when they need to sleep. Melatonin supplements have been shown to improve daytime sleep quality and duration, but not nighttime alertness, in people with shift work disorder. The American Academy of Sleep Medicine recommends that night shift workers with this disorder take melatonin prior to daytime sleep.

INSOMNIA

Melatonin supplements are also used for insomnia. A 2013 analysis of 19 randomized placebo-controlled trials of people with primary sleep disorders found that melatonin slightly improved time to fall asleep, total sleep time, and overall sleep quality. A 2007 study of people ages 55 and up with insomnia found that prolonged-release melatonin significantly improved quality of sleep and morning alertness.

JET LAG

Research has shown that melatonin supplements may help with jet lag. Jet lag is caused by rapid travel across several time zones. Its symptoms include disturbed sleep, daytime fatigue, indigestion, and a general feeling of discomfort. The American Academy of Sleep Medicine supports using melatonin to reduce jet lag symptoms and improve sleep after traveling across more than one time zone. If you're trying to reset your biological clock, take melatonin at local bedtime nightly until you have adapted to the local time at your destination.

MELATONIN SAFETY

Melatonin supplements are generally considered safe when taken short-term. One study found that melatonin supplements might worsen moods in elderly people with dementia. Side effects are uncommon, but can include drowsiness, headache, dizziness, or nausea. Melatonin can interact with anticoagulants, anticonvulsants, birth control pills, immunosuppressants, and diabetes medications.

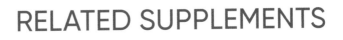

RELATED SUPPLEMENTS

Some dietary supplements contain substances that can be changed into melatonin in the body: L-tryptophan and 5-hydroxytryptophan (5-HTP). These have been researched as sleep aids, but have not been shown to be effective for insomnia. The use of L-tryptophan supplements may be linked to eosinophilia-myalgia syndrome (EMS), a complex, potentially fatal disorder with multiple symptoms including severe muscle pain.

SLEEP FORMULA SUPPLEMENTS

Some "sleep formula" dietary supplements combine ingredients such as melatonin and 5-HTP with herbs such as valerian, hops, lemon balm, passionflower, and kava. There is little evidence on these preparations from studies in people. Plus, kava has been linked to severe liver damage.

CONCERN OVER KAVA

Although the herb kava appears to have sedative effects and may help promote sleep, kava-containing supplements have been linked to a risk of severe liver damage. Also, very little research has been done on whether kava is even helpful for insomnia. It's probably best to avoid kava and products that contain it.

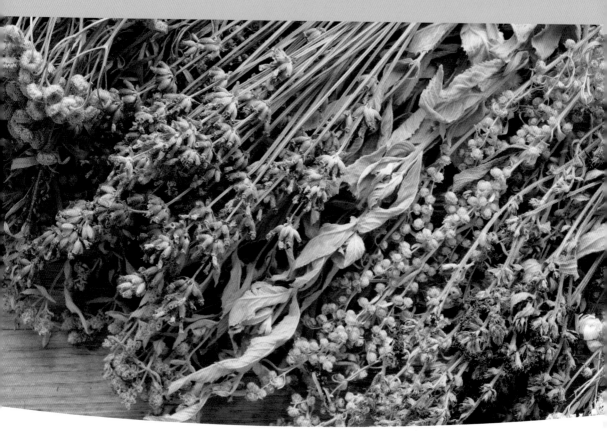

HERBS

Plants have been used as nature's primary medicine for thousands of years. People from every continent have used leaves, stems, seeds, fruits, bark, and roots to enhance healing. Indeed, most modern pharmaceuticals are of plant origin.

A common perception is that because herbs are natural, they are automatically gentler and don't cause side effects like drugs do. That's not always the case, however. Some herbs do have a mild effect and don't appear to cause adverse reactions. But herbal preparations are not as strictly regulated in the United States as are medications, so it's difficult to be sure that you're getting the ingredients and doses that you pay for. In addition, some herbs can cause dangerous side effects, especially when taken at high doses, taken for longer than recommended, or taken while you're using medication.

So, if you are taking any prescription medication, don't take any herbs until you've cleared it with your doctor. If you are taking any over-the-counter medication, it is wise to talk with your pharmacist to ensure there will be no danger in mixing it with your chosen herbs. Some herbal remedies can interact with prescription and over-the-counter medications. And, as an added dose of caution, if you have any chronic medical conditions or any questions about the herbs themselves, talk to a doctor or pharmacist who is experienced in the use of herbs before you attempt herbal treatment.

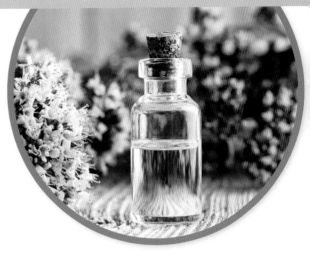

Herbal, or plant-based, remedies can be taken a number of ways. They are available as teas, capsules, tinctures, and liquid extracts for internal use. Some can also be used externally in baths, compresses, or poultices.

There are numerous herbs routinely suggested for treating insomnia. Most of these appear to have a mild sedating effect that may help ease stress and anxiety. The herbs most commonly used to promote sleep are:

- Valerian
- Hops
- Passionflower
- Chamomile
- St. John's wort
- Lemon balm

HERBAL TEAS

There are numerous herbal teas routinely suggested for treating insomnia. Most appear to have a mild sedating effect that may help ease stress and anxiety. You can find the ingredients for making the teas—or the prepackaged teas themselves—at health food stores and even some drugstores and supermarkets. Mix up one or another of the teas (but don't combine them) and drink a cup about 30 minutes before bedtime. (If you're pregnant, don't try herbal tea unless approved by your doctor.)

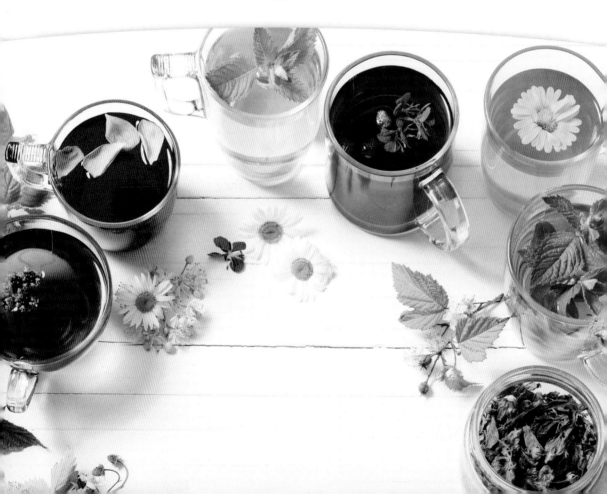

USING HERBS SAFELY

To use herbs safely, you should follow some basic guidelines:

- Follow recommended doses. More does not mean better.
- Stop using a remedy if you experience any side effects.
- Do not collect herbs from the wild.
- Only buy over-the-counter remedies if the packet states what it contains.
- Don't take herbal remedies if you are pregnant or nursing.
- Follow the directions on the package. Most herbal sedatives should be taken 30 to 45 minutes before bedtime.

VALERIAN

Among many herbal medicine proponents, valerian is considered the premier herb to treat insomnia and stress. Some research has suggested that it is an effective relaxant that doesn't cause the drowsiness that often accompanies sedatives. Several studies show that valerian shortens the time needed to fall asleep and improves quality of sleep. Valerian has a disagreeable taste, so mix it with other herbs such as peppermint if you drink it as tea. Take a cup of tea or 2 capsules of the powdered root an hour before bed. Or take ½ to 1 teaspoon (2 to 4 droppers full) of tincture up to three times a day. A tincture is an herb extracted in alcohol, glycerin, or vinegar and sold as liquid drops.

Don't take valerian if you are pregnant, nursing, or taking other sedatives.

HOPS

Aside from being an ingredient in beer, hops are known in Europe for its calming effect and usefulness in treating insomnia. The science supporting this benefit is thin, but the European experience may make it worth a try. For promoting sleep, a typical dose of hops is 2 or 3 capsules or 1 or 2 teaspoons of tincture (an herb extracted in alcohol, glycerin, or vinegar and sold as liquid drops) half an hour before bed. Another option is a bedtime tea. Stir a teaspoon of whole hops into a cup of boiling water, steep 10 minutes, strain, and drink.

CHAMOMILE

Chamomile's sweet, apple-like aroma makes it a favorite tea ingredient. Chamomile has been widely used for centuries to treat stomach upsets and cramps and as a mild sedative that helps promote sleep. While the herb is generally considered quite safe, people who are allergic to ragweed should pass on chamomile. For a soothing nightcap, steep a tablespoon of chamomile in a cup of hot water for 10–15 minutes, strain, and then sip the tea before climbing into bed.

LEMON BALM

Lemon balm, an herb in the mint family, has long been used to remedy insomnia and relieve tension, anxiety, and other nervous disorders. The German Commission E, a scientific group that makes recommendations about herbal therapy to the German government, supports the use of lemon balm as a mild sedative. Lemon balm does not appear to cause adverse effects, and it makes a pleasant-tasting tea. Try a cup of lemon balm tea before bed to see if it helps you sleep tight. Prepare the tea by stirring 2 to 4 teaspoons of the herb into a cup of boiling water; then strain and drink.